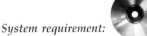

System requirement:

- Windows XP or above
- Power DVD player (software)
- Windows media player 10.0 version or above (software)
- *Accompanying CD ROM is playable only in Computer and not in CD player.*

Chest X-ray Made Easy

D Karthikeyan DMRD DNB
Consultant Radiologist
Bharat Heart Scans
Chennai

Deepa Chegu DMRD
Consultant Radiologist
Bharat Heart Scans
Chennai

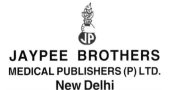

JAYPEE BROTHERS
MEDICAL PUBLISHERS (P) LTD.
New Delhi

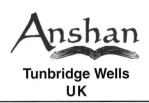

Tunbridge Wells
UK

First published in the UK by

Anshan Ltd
in 2007

6 Newlands Road
Tunbridge Wells
Kent TN4 9AT, UK

Tel: +44 (0)1892 557767
Fax: +44 (0)1892 530358
E-mail: info@anshan.co.uk
www.anshan.co.uk

ISBN 10   1-905740-59-X
ISBN 13   978-1-905740-59-8

British Library Cataloguing in Publication Data
A catalogue record for this book is available from the British Library

Printed in India by Ajanta Offset & Packagings Ltd., New Delhi

PREFACE

Traditionally plain X-ray provides the earliest opportunity in many instances for diagnosing various pathologies of the chest providing a cost effective rapid screening tool. In this era of modern cross-sectional imaging, plain radiograph is often undervalued and the most significant limitation of the Chest X-ray seems to be the lack of interest and experience among the students.

This book tries to present a very easy to use practical approach to Chest X-ray. We hope we can rekindle the interests among medical students and various post-graduates to this simple but powerful diagnostic tool.

D Karthikeyan
Deepa Chegu

Contents

CHAPTER 1

Chest X-ray

INTRODUCTION

Radiology is an indispensable part of clinical medicine. The chest X-ray is the most commonly performed radiographic examination. It is usually recommended as the initial investigation for patients with complaints of shortness of breath, persistent cough, chest pain or a chest injury.

The ability to evaluate and understand this aspect of conventional radiology is critical for medical students entering their clinical years and for physicians throughout their careers.

OBJECTIVES OF CHEST X-RAY

Identify normal cardiothoracic anatomical structures demonstrable on a chest film.

Recognize radiographic signs of lung pathologies like atelectasis, consolidation, pneumothorax, pleural and pericardial effusions, hyperinflation.

Correlate physical signs and symptoms of cardiopulmonary disease with chest radiographic findings.

STANDARD VIEWS

- Posteroanterior (PA)
- Lateral X-ray
- Anteroposterior (AP)

SPECIAL VIEWS

The frontal and lateral projections suffice for most radiographic purposes. Other special views include:

- Lordotic view
- Inspiration and expiration film
- Reverse lordotic view
- Oblique
- Supine (bedside CXR)
- Lateral decubitus film.

High Penetration Film with Moving Grid (Bucky Film)

1. Obesity
2. Dense pleural or pulmonary opacities
3. Calcified lesions
4. Lesions obscured by heart or diaphragms
5. Air bronchograms in densely infiltrated areas.

To show the hidden areas on PA view (mediastinum, hila), rib destruction, cavitation, calcification, airways a penetrated film should be obtained.

Intrathoracic Pressure Maneuvers

1. Valsalva maneuver: shrinks pulmonary vessels
2. Muller maneuver: distends pulmonary vessels.

Indications

a. Distinguish blood vessel from lymph node
b. Distinguish A-V malformation from solid lesion.

Supine Film

Decreases lung volume—highlights infiltrates and interstitium.

Increases venous return to heart—distends azygous vein and pulmonary vein.

Diaphragm rises and intracardiac pressure increases—heart and mediastinal structures enlarge.

Fluid and air migrate.

Pleural effusions disappear.

Small pneumothorax disappears.

Air-fluid levels (e.g. lung abscess) disappear.

Pneumothorax Signs on Supine Film

1. Deep sulcus sign
   a. Costophrenic angle sharply outlined by air
   b. Diaphragm-mediastinal junction sharply outlined
2. Hyperlucency superimposed over liver shadow.

TECHNIQUES

The ideal radiograph provides image of structures within the chest using minimum radiation.

PA VIEW

The standard chest examination consists of a PA (posterioranterior) and lateral chest X-ray.

The patient should be examined in full inspiration.

* Patient's chest is placed against the cassette.
* The PA view minimizes cardiac magnification which can complicate other views.

LATERAL VIEW

A lateral view is ordered in conjunction with a PA view.

Left side of the chest is conventionally placed against the cassette.

Since the right side of the body is closer to the source of the X-rays, the right side is magnified greater than the left side.

This view may expose lesions that are retrosternal or hidden by the diaphragm. The patient is placed with the film against the side of the chest where the lesion is suspected. For example, a left lateral view (with the left side of the chest held against the film) would be used to examine the area behind the left side of the heart. **It is best when the lesion is as close to the film as possible.**

AP VIEW

It is performed on patients who are unable to stand for the PA exam.

Performed at the bedside.

This view may cause cardiac magnification.

AP view is sometimes useful to determine whether a questionable opacity on PA view is genuine by altering the position of overlying ribs. AP view also provides better visualization of posterior chest.

LORDOTIC VIEW

Useful to demonstrate lung apices free from superimposed shadows of clavicle and first rib and middle lobe pathologies like middle lobe collapse/consolidation.

LATERAL DECUBITUS

Helpful to assess the volume of pleural effusion and demonstrate whether a pleural effusion is mobile or loculated. It is a sensitive method for detecting small quantities of pleural fluid (50-100 ml) and also to differentiate between subpulmonic effusion and high diaphragm. Also helps to assess the nondependent hemithorax to confirm a pneumothorax in a patient who could not be examined erect. Additionally, the dependant lung should increase in density due to atelectasis from the weight of the mediastinum putting pressure on it. Failure to do so indicates air trapping.

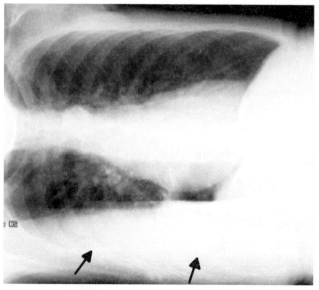

FIGURE 1.1: Lateral decubitus X-ray

PAIRED INSPIRATORY-EXPIRATION VIEW

Films exposed in expiration is important in the investigation of air trapping, e.g. in cases of foreign body aspiration. An expiratory film is also helpful to demonstrate small pneumothorax. Diaphragmatic function is also well-assessed on expiratory films.

OBLIQUE VIEW

Useful to demonstrate pleural plaques, chest wall lesions, rib lesions and lower lobe collapse.

TECHNICAL CONSIDERATIONS

Inspiration

The patient should be examined in full inspiration. This greatly helps the radiologist to determine if there are intrapulmonary abnormalities. The diaphragm should be found at about the level of the 8th-10th posterior rib or 5th-6th anterior rib on good inspiration.

Penetration

Adequate penetration of the patient by radiation is also required for a good film. On a good PA film, the thoracic spine disk spaces should be barely visible through the heart but bony details of the spine are not usually seen. On the other hand penetration is sufficient that broncho-vascular structures can usually be seen through the heart.

On the lateral view, you can look for proper penetration and inspiration by observing that the spine appears to darken as you move caudally. This is due to more air

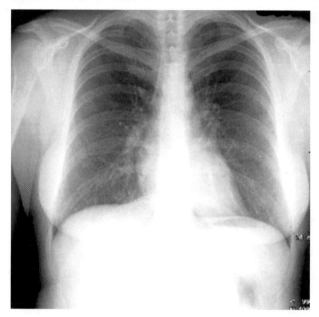

FIGURE 1.2: PA view in good inspiration

in lung in the lower lobes and less chest wall. The sternum should be seen edge on and posteriorly you should see two sets of ribs.

Rotation

The technologists are usually very careful to X-ray the patient flat against the cassette. If there is rotation of the patient, the mediastinum may look very unusual. One can access patient rotation by observing the clavicular heads and determining whether they are in equal distance from the spinous process of the thoracic vertebral bodies.

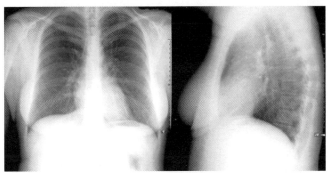

FIGURES 1.3A and B: Normal PA and lateral chest X-ray

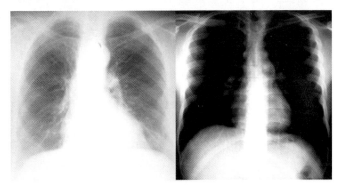

FIGURES 1.4A and B

UNDERPENETRATED   OVERPENETRATED

- Lung fields are "blacker" than usual
- There is no adequate lung detail
- Absence of peripheral vasculature
- See vertebrae extending down into the abdominal region

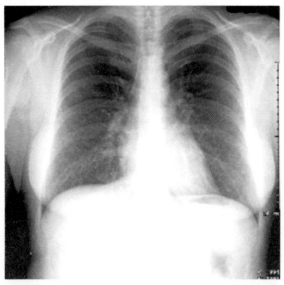

FIGURE 1.5: Normal PA film without any rotation

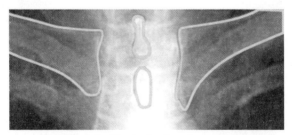

FIGURE 1.6: Clavicular head and spinous process alignment showing a straight film

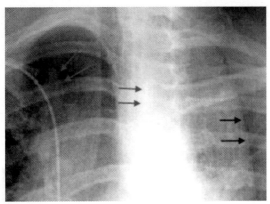

FIGURE 1.7: Rotated film. Note the positioning of the heads of the clavicles (black arrows) and the spinous processes.

NORMAL ANATOMY

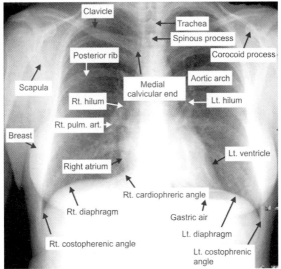

FIGURE 1.8: Normal structures

LUNG ZONES

BRONCHOPULMONARY SEGMENTS

Each bronchial division and its accompanying pulmonary arterial branch supply a particular region of lung. This entire unit of lung is called **BRONCHOPULMONARY SEGMENT**. Each segment is pyramidal shaped with apex towards hilum. They are functional independent respiratory units.

RIGHT LUNG has two fissures (minor and major) dividing the lung into 3 lobes—upper, middle, lower.

Bronchopulmonary segments in right lung (10 segments).

UPPER LOBE	*MIDDLE LOBE*	*LOWER LOBE*
APICAL	MEDIAL	APICAL
ANTERIOR	LATERAL	ANTERIOR BASAL
POSTERIOR		POSTERIOR BASAL
		MEDIAL BASAL
		LATERAL BASAL

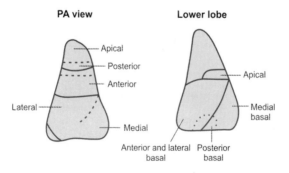

FIGURE 1.9: PA view

Lateral view

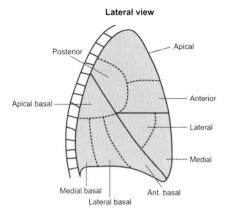

FIGURE 1.10: Lateral view

LEFT LUNG has 1 fissure (major) dividing the lung into 2 lobes—upper (includes lingual) and lower.

Bronchopulmonary segments in left lung (8 segemnts)

UPPER LOBE	*LINGULA*	*LOWER LOBE*
APICOPOSTERIOR	SUPERIOR	APICAL
ANTERIOR	INFERIOR	ANTERIOR BASAL
		LATERAL BASAL
		POSTERIOR BASAL

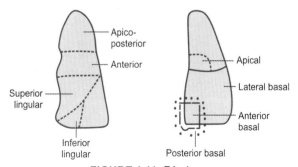

FIGURE 1.11: PA view

Lateral view

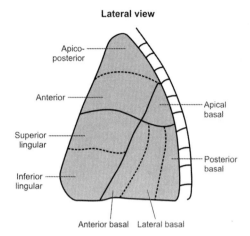

FIGURE 1.12: Lateral view

Extent of Lobes on Normal Films

These diagrams show the extent of the lobes in a normal subject, as seen on the PA and lateral films.

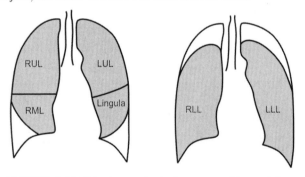

FIGURE 1.13: PA view: extent of upper and lower lobes. Note the extensive overlap. The lower lobes extend considerably higher than many realise

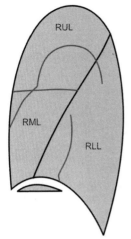
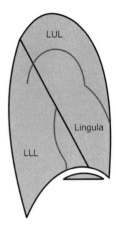

FIGURE 1.14: Lateral view: extent of lobes on the lateral view (note that the left and right sides are in practice superimposed upon one another)

FISSURES

Fissures can be visualized only when the X-ray beam is tangential.

On the PA chest X-ray, the minor fissure divides the right middle lobe from the right upper lobe and is sometimes not well seen. There is no minor fissure on the left. It runs from the hilum to the region of sixth rib in the axillary line. Often this fissure is incomplete and runs anteriorly and slightly downwards.

The major fissures are usually not well seen on the PA view because you are looking through them obliquely. If there is fluid in the fissure, it is occasionally manifested as a density at the lower lateral margin. Both major fissures start posteriorly at the level T4/T5 and passes through the hilum. The left is steeper and ends 5 cm behind the anterior costophrenic angle and the the right major fissure ends just behind the costophrenic angle.

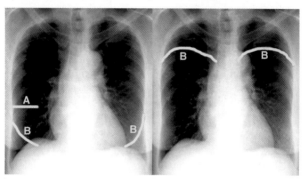

FIGURE 1.15: Right minor fissure (A), borders (B) of the major fissures bilaterally. Superior border of the major. Inferior fissures (B) bilaterally

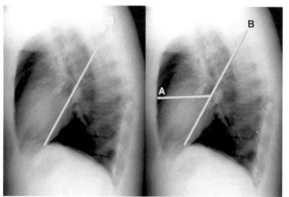

FIGURE 1.16: On the lateral view, both lungs are superimposed. The left lung has only a major fissure (B). The right lung will have both the major(B) and minor fissure(A)

Accessory Fissures

1. Azygos fissure: Comma shaped. Usually seen in the apex of right lung. It contains paired folds of parietal and visceral pleura with the azygos vein which has failed to migrate normally.
2. Left-sided minor fissure: Separates lingual from other upper lobe segments.

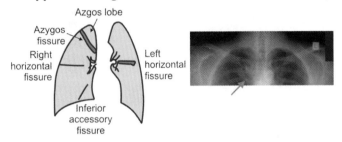

FIGURE 1.17: Chest X-ray showing azygos fissure

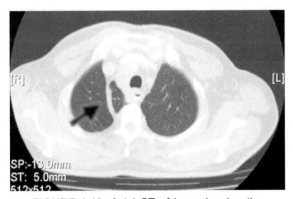

FIGURE 1.18: Axial CT of lung showing the azygos fissure

3. Superior accessory fissure: Common on right side (in 5% of population). On PA view it resembles minor fissure and separates apical from basal segments of lower lobe. On lateral view this fissure is seen to run posteriorly from the hilum.

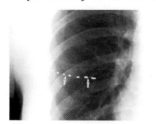 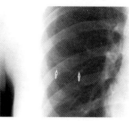

FIGURES 1.19A and B: CXR showing the course of the superior accessory fissure

4. Inferior accessory fissure: Common on the right side and runs up from cardiophrenic angle obliquely. Usually separates medial basal sement from the rest of the basal segments.

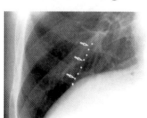 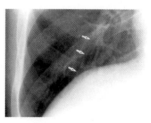

FIGURES 1.20A AND B: CXR showing the course of the inferior accessory fissure

Major Oblique Fissure	Separates the LUL from the LLL
Right Major Fissure	Separates the RUL/RML from the RLL
Right Minor Fissure	Separates the RUL from the RML

MEDIASTINUM AND HEART

Mediastinum separates the thoracic cavity into right and left pleural spaces. It extends from thoracic inlet to the diaphragm and is enveloped by parietal pleura. It extends anteriorly to the sternum and posteriorly to paravertebral gutters.

Central dense shadow on PA view consists of mediastinum, spine sternum.

Division of Mediastinum

Conventional Method

Mediastinum is conventionally divided into superior, anterior, middle and posterior compartments.

Superior mediastinum: Extends from thoracic inlet superiorly to an imaginary line joining sternal angle and 4th intervertebral disk space inferiorly.

Anterior medistinum: Space bounded by sternum anteriorly and posteriorly by pericardium.

Middle mediastinum: Space containing pericardium and contents, trachea, vena cava.

Posterior mediastinum: Space posterior to pericardium upto paravertebral gutters.

Felson's Method

In this method, anterior mediastinum includes the space anterior to the line drawn along the posterior margin of pericardium and anterior to the trachea. This space includes the heart.

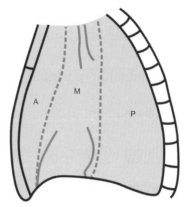

FIGURE 1.21: Schematic showing the division of mediastinum A=anterior: M=middle: P= posterior

Middle mediastinum includes trachea and all structures anterior to a line drawn 1 cm posterior to the anterior border of vertebral body.

Posterior mediastinum includes paravertebral gutters.

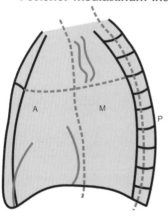

FIGURE 1.22: A = anterior mediastinum, M =middle mediastinum, P = posterior mediastinum

Other methods: Sutton's method, Heitzman's method.

- Two-thirds of the heart lies on the left side of the chest, with one-third on the right. The heart should take up no more than half of the thoracic cavity.

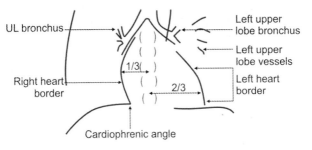

FIGURE 1.23

- The left border of the heart is made up by the left atrium and left ventricle.
- The right border is made up by the right atrium alone. Above the right heart border lies the edge of the superior vena cava. The right ventricle sits anteriorly and therefore does not have a border on the PA chest X-ray film.
- On a lateral chest X-ray, the heart lies antero-inferiorly.
- Apparent cardiac enlargement occurs with short FFD, on expiration, in AP and supine views.

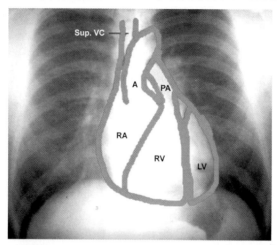

FIGURE 1.24: PA view

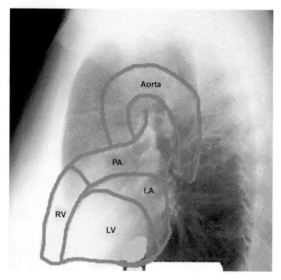

FIGURE 1.25: Lateral view

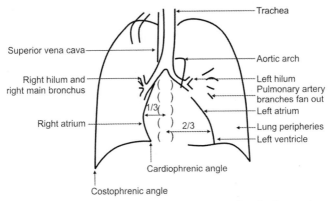

FIGURE 1.26: Structures forming the mediastinal margins

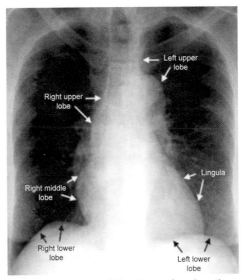

FIGURE 1.27: The lobes of the lungs forming the margins of the lungs along the mediastinum and chest wall

Hila

The "hilum" is composed of the pulmonary artery and its branches, and adjacent airway and pulmonary veins. Since airways do not produce a significant shadow on plain film radiography, the majority of the detectable "hilar" structures are vascular.

The pulmonary arteries and upper lobe veins significantly contribute to the hilar shadow on plain chest X-ray.

Left hilum is slightly at a higher position (0.5-2 cm) than the right hilum. Both the hila should be of equal size, density with concave lateral borders. Normal lymph nodes are not seen.

The right pulmonary artery courses below the level of left main stem bronchus. As a result, the right hilar shadow is inferior to the left on the PA projection. This is seen in 70% of the population. In the rest of the 30%, the hilar shadows are equal in height.

The right pulmonary artery is approximately 3 times larger than the LPA.

On the lateral projection, the right hilum is anterior to a line drawn through the tracheal air column.

Pulmonary Vessels

The arteries and veins branch out from the hila, becoming smaller towards the periphery. The larger central vessels are better seen; peripherally the vessels overlap as they run laterally.

In the upright position, the lower lung vessels are larger than the upper lung vessels, due to gravitational effects on flow. If the patient is supine, there is redistribution (increase) in flow to the upper lung vessels. This is called **cephalization** of flow. Congestive heart failure also causes redistribution to the upper lung vessels, even when the patient is upright when the X-ray film is taken.

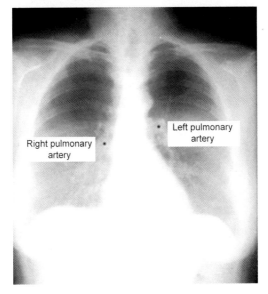

Left pulmonary artery

Right pulmonary artery

FIGURE 1.28: Pulmonary arteries

On the left side, the left pulmonary artery is directed posterolaterally, towards the left scapula. This artery goes over the left main stem bronchus, and therefore, the left pulmonary artery is located higher than the right pulmonary artery. On the lateral projection, the left pulmonary artery is posterior to a line drawn down the tracheal air column.

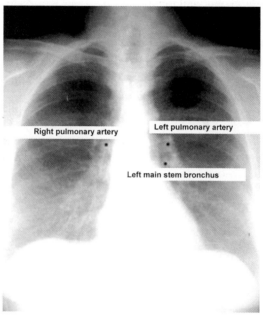

FIGURE 1.29: Relationship of artery and bronchus

DIAPHRAGM

Diaphragm is a dome-shaped musculotendinous partition that separates thoracic cavity from abdominal cavity. It is formed by fusion of septum transversum, dorsal mesogastrium, pleuroperitoneal folds and side wall mesenchyme.

It has sternal, costal and vertebral origin.

It consists of a central tendon, with right and left leaflets composed of striated muscles. Three large openings disrupt the continuity of the diaphragm: the aortic, esophageal, and inferior vena caval apertures. The diaphragm is covered by parietal pleura and peritoneum except for the bare area of the liver. Anatomically, the diaphragm is composed of two parts: the lumbar diaphragm and costal diaphragm.

Diaphragm has smooth outline in most individuals. Angle of contact with the chest wall is acute and sharp. Blunting of the angle is sometimes normally seen in athletes. Normally right hemidiaphragm is 1.5-2.5 cm higher than the left and is usually at the level of 6th rib anteriorly. Difference of more than 3 cm is considered abnormal. In 3% of population, left hemidiaphragm is at a higher level than the right.

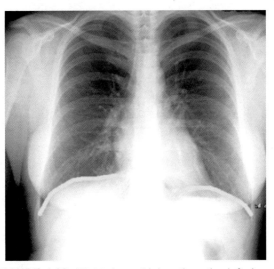

FIGURE 1.30: Right dome higher than the left dome

Normal excursion of the diaphragm is between 1.5 and 2.5 cm.

Check for flattening of dome of diaphragm by drawing a line perpendicular from the mid point of the dome to a line joining costophrenic and cardiophrenic angles. This distance is usually >1.5 cm if it is less than 1.5 cm, then it is considered flattened.

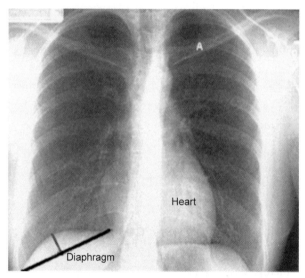

FIGURE 1.31: CXR showing the method of measuring the dome

Check for the presence of the gastric gas bubble below the left hemidiaphragm.

Look below the diaphragm for any evidence of free air.

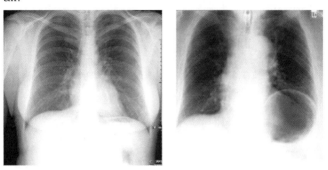

FIGURES 1.32A and B: (A) Normal (B) Large gastric bubble

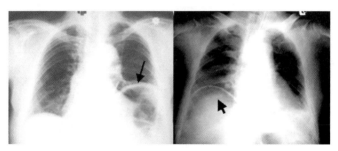

FIGURES 1.33A and B: (A) Eventration of left hemi-diaphragm (B) Air under the diaphragm

NORMAL VARIANTS

1. Scalloping
2. Muscle slips
3. Diaphragmatic humps and dromedary diaphragm
4. Eventration
5. Accessory diaphragm

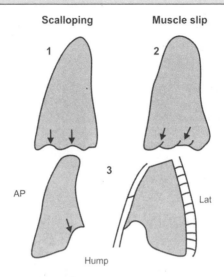

FIGURE 1.34: Diaphragmatic contours

INTERPRETATION: *How to look at a Chest PA view*

COMPARISON WITH PREVIOUS X-RAYS

This is often the single most important diagnostic maneuver in the interpretation of chest roentgenograms. Every effort should be made to obtain previous films for comparison with the current films.

The easiest way to identify a new abnormality is to note its absence on a previous film!!

The key to successfully interpreting any radiograph is to be systematic.

Examine all parts of the film in an orderly manner, and do this consistently.

Identification

1. Correct patient
2. Correct date and time
3. Correct examination.

Side Marker

The position of side marker allows the radiograph to be oriented correctly for reading.

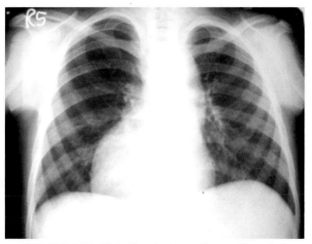

FIGURE 1.35: Note the dextrocardia, easily noted if the side marker is placed correctly

Technique

Next concentrate on the technical factors:

1. Is the examination complete?
2. Are all the requested views included?

3. Is the entire anatomical area included on the films?
   a. Projection
   b. Position
   c. Penetration
   d. Rotation
   e. inspiration.

Systematic Analysis

1. Soft tissue including breast, chest wall, companion shadow
2. Bones—shoulder girdles, spine and rib cage
3. Diaphragm position, shape, subdiaphragmatic abnormalities
4. Review abdomen for bowel gas, organ size, abnormal calcifications, free air
5. Plastic – ETT, lines, tubes
6. Review mediastinum:
   a. Overall size and shape
   b. Trachea: position, carina. The trachea should be central
   c. Margins: SVC, ascending aorta, right atrium, left subclavian artery, aortic arch, main pulmonary artery, left ventricle
   d. Lines and stripes: paratracheal, paraspinal, paraesophageal (azygoesophageal), para-aortic
   e. Retrosternal clear space
7. Heart size, shape: The width of the heart should be no greater than 50% of the width of the rib cage

8. Review hila:
   a. Normal relationships
   b. Size
9. Parenchyma: Now finally ready to examine the lungs!! Mentally divide the entire chest into upper, middle and lower thirds. Then, methodically compare the right and left sides of each lung section looking for asymmetry. The easiest way to identify an abnormality is to confirm that it does not exist on the other side!!

   Compare lung sizes, aeration, vascular distinctness, and abnormal opacities.
10. Pleura: Costophrenic and cardiophrenic angles, thickening fissures—major and minor—if seen.

HIDDEN AREAS

- Supraclavicular regions
- Ends of ribs
- Retroclavicular regions
- Posterior mediastinal and paravertebral regions.

How to Read a Lateral Film

When reading a patient's chest films you should look at both the PA and the lateral films.

Lateral chest X-ray can be taken with either the right or left side of the patient against the film.

Mount the film in such way that the vertebral column is on the right of you and the front of the chest is on the left of you, as shown in Figure 1.38.

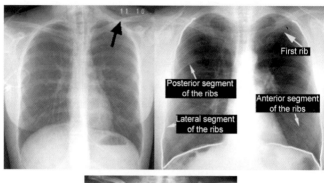

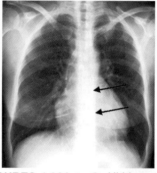

FIGURES 1.36A to C: Hidden areas

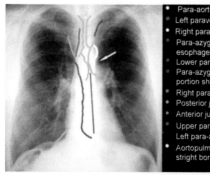

- Para-aortic line
- Left paravertebral line (6 to 15 mm wide)
- Right paravertebral line (2 to 4 mm wide)
- Para-azygo-esophageal line (pleuro-esophageal line)
- Lower paravenous line (LVC)
- Para-azygo-esophageal line (upper portion should be concave)
- Right paratracheal stripe (max 5 mm)
- Posterior junction line
- Anterior junction line
- Upper paravenous line (SVC or RBCV)
- Left para-arterial line (LSCA)
- Aortopulmonary window (concave or stright border, nerve convex)

FIGURES 1.37A and B: Mediastinal lines

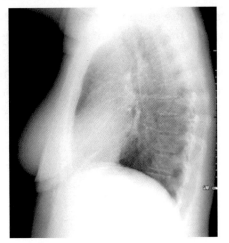

FIGURE 1.38: Lateral X-ray

Identify the Diaphragms

Right diaphragm can be seen to stretch across the whole thorax and can be seen clearly through the heart. Left diaphragm seems to disappear when it reaches the posterior border of heart. Gastric air bubble is seen closer to the left diaphragm. Posterior costophrenic angles are acute. Small amount of pleural fluid can blunt the CP angle.

Vertebral Translucency

Vertebral bodies become more translucent (darker) caudally. Loss of this translucency may be a sign of posterior basal segment pathology. Check the size, shape and density of vertebrae.

Compare the appearance of lung fields in front of and above the heart to those behind. They should be of equal density.

Look carefully at the clear spaces: retrosternal and retrocardiac spaces. These are areas of increased translucency corresponding to the site where both the lungs meet. Loss of translucency indicates pathology.

Normal retrosternal space measures 3 cm at its widest point. Retrosternal space obliterated in anterior mediastinal masses. Retrosternal space is widened in emphysema.

Check the position of fissures – horizontal and oblique fissure. Displacement, thickening of fissures has to noted. Look for interlobar effusions.

Check the density of hila.

Trachea is seen to pass down in posterior direction to T6-T7 level. Posterior tracheal wall measures less than 5 mm (which includes tracheal and esophageal wall).

Soft tissues and bones have to studied. Sternum and scapulae are well seen.

SILHOUETTE SIGN

One of the most useful signs in chest radiology is the silhouette sign. This was described by Dr Ben Felson. The silhouette sign is actually elimination of the silhouette or loss of lung/soft tissue interface caused by a mass or fluid in the normally air filled lung. For example, if an intrathoracic opacity is in anatomic contact with the heart border, then the opacity will obscure that border. The sign is commonly applied to the heart, aorta, chest wall, and diaphragm. ***The location of this abnormality can help to determine the location anatomically.***

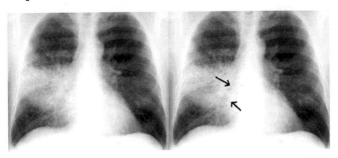

FIGURE 1.39: The right heart border is silhouetted out. This is caused by a pneumonia, involving the Rt. middle lobe.

Silhouette/Structure	Contact with Lung
Upper right heart border/ascending aorta	Anterior segment of RUL
Right heart border	RML (medial)
Upper left heart border	Anterior segment of LUL
Left heart border	Lingula (anterior)
Aortic knob	Apical portion of LUL (posterior)
Anterior hemidiaphragms	Lower lobes (anterior)

Loss of right heart border
1. Right middle lobe ateletctasis or airspace consolidation
2. Pleural disease
3. Mediastinal disease
4. Pectus excavatum
5. Scimitar syndrome

Loss of aortic knob
1. Left upper lobe disease
2. Mediastinal disease
3. Pleural disease

Loss of left heart border
1. Lingular collapse or airspace consolidation
2. Pleural disease
3. Mediastinal disease
4. Pericardial fat

Loss of hemidiaphragm
1. Lower lobe disease
2. Pleural disease

AIR BRONCHOGRAM

- Air bronchogram is a tubular outline of an airway made visible by filling of the surrounding alveoli by fluid or inflammatory exudates.
- It is diagnostic of consolidation.

Normal bronchi not usually visualized due to thin walls and an air-air interface.

Causes of air bronchograms are; consolidation, pulmonary edema, nonobstructive pulmonary atelectasis, severe interstitial disease, neoplasm and normal expiration.

CONSOLIDATION

Consolidation is defined as a process in which air in the alveoli is replaced by products of disease. The bronchi to the consolidated area are usually widely patent. In most

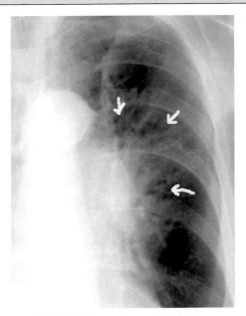

FIGURE 1.40: Air bronchograms

instances, alveolar filling is patchy, i.e. not all acini are involved. The radiographic opacity is therefore nonhomogeneous, sometimes with air bronchogram. Causes include:

- Pus: bacterial pneumonia
- Blood: contusion, pulmonary hemorrhage
- Water: pulmonary alveolar edema, aspiration
- Cells: lymphoma, bronchioloalveolar cell carcinoma
- Protein: pulmonary alveolar proteinosis

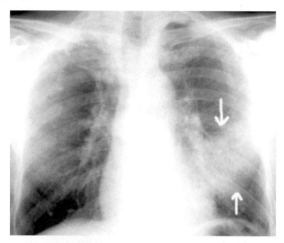

FIGURE 1.41: Consolidation

COLLAPSE (ATELECTASIS)

Atelectasis is volume loss due to alveolar collapse or failure to expand causing increased opacification of radiograph. Collapse may affect a whole lung or a subdivision (lobe, segment).

Types

- Obstructive
- Compressive
- Cicatrization
- Adhesive
- Passive.

General Features of Lobar Collapse

- Shift of fissures

- Area of increased opacity
- Crowding of vessels
- Tracheal displacement towards the side of the collapse
- Hilar shift
- Mediastinal shift towards the side of the collapse
- Elevation of the hemidiaphragm
- Herniation of the opposite lung across the midline.

Other Signs

- A hilar mass, which also suggests carcinoma as the cause.
- The presence of a foreign body.
- The presence of an endotracheal tube; is it sited too low?
- Other evidence of malignant disease (e.g. rib metastases, effusion).

Collapse of Individual Lobes

Right Upper Lobe Collapse

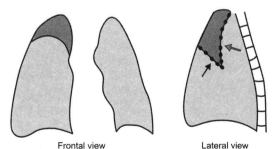

Frontal view   Lateral view

FIGURE 1.42: The minor and major fissures move towards each other (black arrow=minor, white arrow=major)

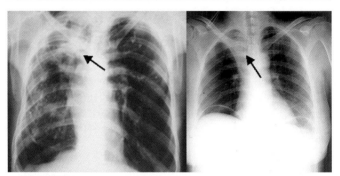

FIGURE 1.43: Examples of right upper lobe collapse

Signs of Right Upper Lobe Collase

- Minor fissure moves upwards with concavity inferiorly
- An area of opacity that lies against apex of mediastinum
- Tracheal shift to the right
- Right hilum is elevated and the intermediate bronchus assumes horizontal position
- Loss of right paratracheal stripe (silhouette sign)

Right Middle Lobe Collapse

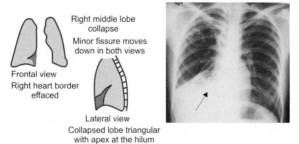

FIGURE 1.44: Example of right middle lobe collapse

Signs of Right Middle Lobe Collapse

- This is often not immediately obvious on the frontal film
- Ill defined shadowing is evident adjacent to the right heart border, which becomes indistinct
- Right heart border is silhouetted
- Minor fissure moves downward
- **Collapse of right middle lobe more obvious on lateral view**
- In lateral view, collapsed lobe has triangular shape with apex at the hilum
- Also best seen in lordotic view.

Right Lower Lobe Collapse

Right lower zone shadowing is combined with obliteration of the hemidiaphragm (silhouette sign). The right heart border, which is anterior, is usually still clearly seen (silhouette sign again). The oblique fissure lies more

Right lower lobe collapse

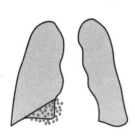
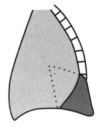

Frontal view   Lateral view

FIGURE 1.45: Opacity in the post costophrenic angle. Major fissure moves backwards

horizontally and may become visible, giving a sharp upper margin to the shadowing. If the lobe collapses completely, it may appear as a triangular opacity behind the right heart border. The heart border, being anterior will still be clearly seen. On the lateral film there is abnormally increased density over the lower thoracic spine due to the triangular opacity of the collapsed lobe.

Left Upper Lobe Collapse

The left lung lacks a middle lobe and therefore a minor fissure, so left upper lobe atelectasis presents a different picture from that of the right upper lobe collapse. The result is predominantly anterior shift of the upper lobe in left upper lobe collapse, with loss of the left upper cardiac border. It casts a veil like opacity over the left hemithorax, normally more dense towards the apex.

Left upper lobe collapse

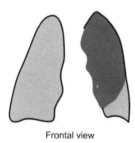

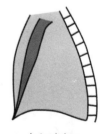

Frontal view

Veil like opacity spreads
from hilum

Lateral view

Major fissure moves forward.
Retrosternal lucency is seen
due to herniated right lung

FIGURE 1.46

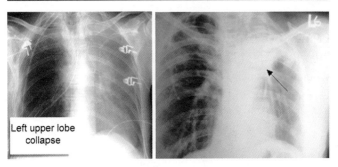

FIGURE 1.47: Examples of left upper lobe collapse

The expanded lower lobe will migrate to a location both superior and posterior to the upper lobe in order to occupy the vacated space and so the aortic knuckle characteristically remains clearly visible.

Left Lower Lobe Collapse

The left lower lobe collapses medially and posteriorly to lie behind the heart. It classically displays a triangular

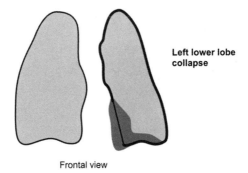

Left lower lobe collapse

Frontal view

FIGURE 1.48

opacity which may be visible through the cardiac shadow, or may overlie it, giving the heart an unusually straight lateral border. The hemidiaphragm may be obscured where the opacity lies against it. On the lateral film there is abnormally increased density over the lower thoracic spine due to the triangular opacity of the collapsed lobe.

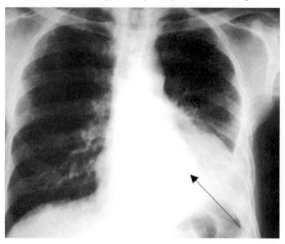

FIGURE 1.49: Left lower lobe collapse

Total Collapse of Lung

Total collapse of a lung occurs when the obstruction is within the main stem bronchus. The appearance is one of total opacification of the affected hemithorax. The volume loss causes deviation of the trachea and shift of the mediastinum to the affected side. Sometimes the opposite lung may herniate across the midline, giving rise to the impression that some lung remains aerated. This

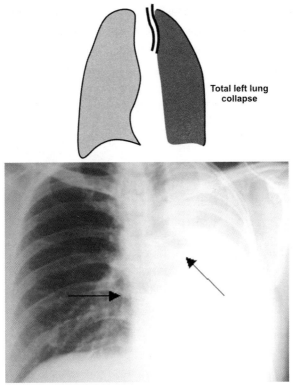

Total left lung collapse

FIGURES 1.50A and B: Total collapse of left lung

is particularily so at the apices, at the site of the anterior and posterior junctional lines. An effusion will produce midline shift in the opposite direction. However, collapse and effusion often coexist, in which case there may be minimal shift.

Segmental atelectasis — Appears as a wedge-shaped opacity with its apex at the hilum and its base in contact with the pleura. Other important features are fissural shift and positive silhouette sign. Sometimes it just appears as a narrow band of opacity.

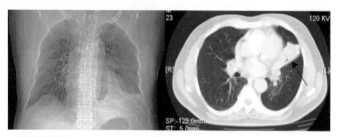

FIGURES 1.51A and B: Digital scanogram and axial CT showing superior lingular segmental atelectasis

Discoid atelectasis — Horizontal linear densities at the lung bases which usually make contact with the pleura. Associated with hypoventilation due to various causes. It's a common form of non-obstructive collapse.

Rounded atelectasis(RA)—It is a form of non-segmental peripheral pulmonary collapse that produces a pleural-based mass-like lesion. It is strongly associated with asbestos exposure. It is about 3-5 cm and is commonly located basally and dorsally and is composed of swirl of atelectatic parenchyma adjacent to thickened pleura. Other names are Blesovky's syndrome, helical atelectasis, pseudotumor, folded lung. Conventional radiography may demonstrate rounded/oval subpleural opacity with vessels and airways converging towards the opacity in a helical fashion producing ***comet tail*** appearance.

RA usually remains stable on serial radiologic studies, although very slow growth or regression may occur.

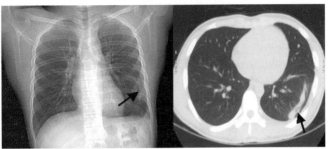

FIGURES 1.52A and B: Digital scanogram and axial CT showing subpleural atelectasis with incurving of broncho-vascular bundle

Major differentiating factors between atelectasis and pneumonia

Atelectasis	Pneumonia
Volume loss	Normal or increased volume
Associated ipsilateral shift	No shift, or if present then contralateral
Linear, wedge-shaped	Consolidation, air space process
Apex at hilum	Not centered at hilum
Air bronchograms can occur in both	

PLEURAL DISEASE

Pleural Effusion

A pleural effusion is defined as fluid accumulating in the pleural space. The pleural space is a potential space lined by the visceral and parietal pleura. Normally less than

5 ml of free fluid is present in the pleural space. Excess pleural fluid accumulates when 1. capillary hydrostatic pressure increases, 2. blood oncotic pressure is low, 3. capillary permeability is increased, and 4. lymphatic obstruction.

The fluid can be transudative or exudative in nature. Terms used to refer to the various nature of effusions include:

- Hydrothorax: transudative effusion, i.e. CHF, hypo-albuminemia
- Pyothorax: pus in the pleural space, i.e. empyema from pneumonia
- Hemothorax: blood
- Chylothorax: chyle.

Malignant Effusion

Bilateral pleural effusions are usually transudates as they develop secondary to generalized systemic problems. Some of the bilateral effusions are exudates and are seen in metastatic disease, rheumatoid disease, lymphoma, SLE. Right-sided effusions are usually associated with ascites, heart failure, liver abscess. Left-sided effusions usually occur with pancreatitis. pericarditis, aortic dissection.

Radiological Signs of Pleural Effusion

The standard posterior-anterior (PA) and lateral chest radiographs remain the most important initial techniques for evaluating the pleural effusion. If fluid is free to distribute itself as influenced by gravity and elastic recoil of the lung, it will collect in the inferior hemithorax and between the inferior surface of the lung and the hemidiaphragm. Small effusions may fail to be detected because of the fluid's position in the posterior costophrenic gutters.

The standard PA radiograph can show changes with effusions as small as 250 ml. The lateral decubitus can sometimes distinguish very small effusions (15-25 ml). An effusion of 1 L will obscure the hemidiaphragm and extend up one-third to one-half of the hemithorax. As much as 200 to 300 ml may only cause blunting of the costophrenic angle laterally on the PA film.

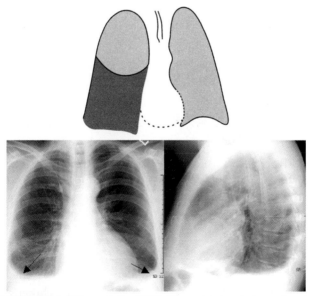

FIGURES 1.53A and B: CXR PA and lateral view showing bilateral pleural effusion. Note the blunting of CP angles with lateralization of the dome

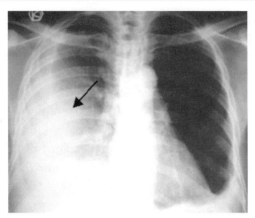

FIGURE 1.54: CXR showing moderate right pleural effusion with mild left pleural effusion

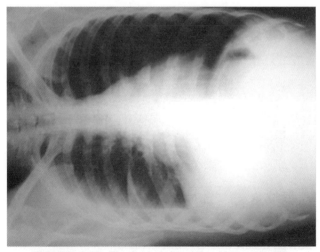

FIGURE 1.55: The lateral decubitus X-ray uses the effect of gravity to help confirm the presence of free-flowing pleural fluid, especially small effusions

Larger effusions take on a typical pattern of (1) homogeneous opacity over the lower hemithorax, (2) obscuration of the hemidiaphragm, and (3) concave upward border with the highest point along the lateral chest wall (meniscus).

Massive effusions cause opacification of hemithorax with shift of the mediastinum to the opposite side and sometimes inversion of ipsilateral diaphragm. Absence of mediastinal shift usually implies obstructive collapse of ipsilateral lung or pleural malignancy.

Causes of Opaque Hemithorax

• Pleural effusion
• Consolidation

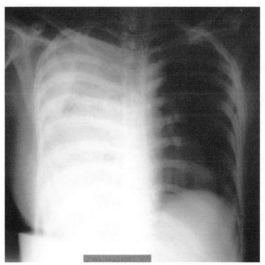

FIGURE 1.56: Causes of opaque right hemithorax

- Collapse
- Massive tumor
- Fibrothorax
- Combination of above lesions
- Lung agenesis
- Pneumonectomy

Pleural Effusions in Supine Patient

Pleural effusions may also accumulate in the pleural space in an "atypical" distribution.

Subpulmonic Effusion

Initially when there is minimal free pleural fluid, it will collect in the inferior hemithorax between the inferior surface of the lung and the hemidiaphragm. It will appear as an elevated hemidiaphragm with an unsual contour that peaks more laterally than usual and has a straight medial segment. A lateral decubitus X-ray is also valuable for confirming the presence of subpulmonic effusions. Left-sided subpulmonic effusions show increased separation between stomach gas and the hemidiaphragm.

Loculated Effusion

Fluid at times becomes loculated in areas of the pleural space.

Fluid can loculate between visceral pleural layers in fissures or also between visceral and parietal layers of pleura.

Phantom tumor refers to fissural loculation of fluid, which commonly occurs in heart failure. These disappear with treatment and recur in the same place on repeated occasions.

Effusion can get loculated against chest wall, appearing as localized opacity convex to the lung with sharp edges.

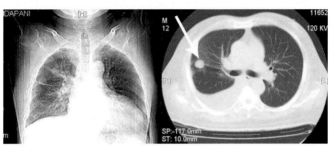

FIGURES 1.57A and B: Loculated effusion in the light minor fissure (arrow)

Lamellar Effusion

In this the fluid gets collected between the lung and visceral pleura. It commonly occurs in cardiac failure. It is seen as a thin band of opacity between the lung and chest wall just above the costophrenic angle and is associated with septal lines.

Causes of Pleural Effusion

Transudate

- Congestive heart failure
- Renal failure
- Nephrotic syndrome
- Cirrhosis

- SVC syndrome
- Meig syndrome

Exudate
- Infection
- Neoplasia
- Pulmonary infarction
- Intra-abdominal process
- Collagen vascular diseases

Hemorrhagic
- Neoplasia
- Tuberculosis
- Pulmonary infarction
- Trauma
- Iatrogenic

Empyema
- Pleural effusion with loculation.

The AP supine film is obtained when the patient is too ill for a standard PA and lateral exposure. It is much less than ideal.

Pneumothorax

When air enters the pleural space, it is termed as pneumo-thorax. The *two major categories* are *spontaneous pneumothoraces* and *traumatic* which develop after trauma. The spontaneous group is further divided into primary and secondary and the traumatic into iatrogenic and non-iatrogenic.

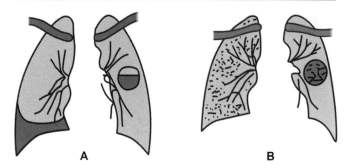

FIGURES 1.58A and B: Comparison of upright and supine films. **A.** Upright PA chest film. Note the pleural effusion in the right hemithorax and the cavitary lesion with an air-fluid interface in the left lung. **B.** Supine AP film, same subject. Note the changes in clavicular position, diaphragmatic height, mediastinal width, and distribution of blood flow. The pleural effusion now appears as a diffuse haziness on the right, and the cavitary lesion no longer shows the air-fluid interface

Primary spontaneous pneumothorax (PSP): The mechanism is felt to be the rupture of subpleural blebs in the lung, usually at the apices. The patients are usually male smokers who are tall and thin. Chest pain and dyspnea are the usual complaints and they are normally not a life-threatening occurrence. PSP occurs predominantly in young adults between 20-40 years.

Secondary spontaneous pneumothorax: There are many associated diseases, but chronic obstructive pulmonary disease and tuberculosis are the common causes.

Non-iatrogenic traumatic pneumothoraces are due to a variety of modes of injuries.

Iatrogenic causes relate to invasive procedures and mechanical ventilation.

Catamenial pneumothorax is commonly a manifestation of endometriosis and is seen in women in their fourth decade. In these cases, pneumothoraces is recurrent occurring in relation to the menses and is predominantly right-sided and small.

Typical signs of pneumothorax on an erect X-ray are:
Pneumothorax is seen as an area of transradiant zone without lung markings in the least dependant part of the chest. The visceral pleural line gets separated from the chest wall and is seen as white line of the pleura. In an upright film this is most likely seen in the apices. Lateral decubitus and expiratory film are helpful to diagnose small pneumothaorax.

Partially collapsed lung may reveal clue to underlying cause of secondary pneumothorax and in primary pneumothorax the small apical blebs can be seen sometimes.

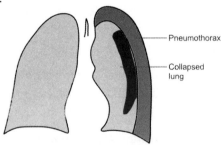

— Pneumothorax

— Collapsed lung

FIGURE 1.59A: Schematic depicting the effects of pneumothorax

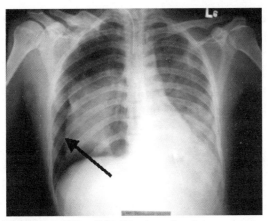

FIGURE 1.59B: CXR PA view showing moderate
right pneumothorax with collapse of right lung

Atypical Signs

It can be difficult to see when the patient is in a supine
position.

When the patient is in supine position air rises anteriorly
and particularly to the medial aspect of the lung and
may be seen as a lucency along the mediastinum. It may
also collect in the inferior sulci causing a deep sulcus sign.

Signs that suggest pneumothorax in these conditions
are: 1. Ipsilateral transradiancy, 2. deep finger like
costophrenic sulcus laterally, 3. anterior costophrenic
recess seen as oblique line mimicking the adjacent
diaphragm "double diaphragm sign", 4. transradiant
band against diaphragm and mediastinal border, and
5. visualization of undersurface of heart and cardiac fat
pads.

Hydropneumothorax: A hydropneumothorax is both air and fluid in the pleural space. It is characterized by an air-fluid level on an upright or decubitus film in a patient with a pneumothorax. Some causes of a hydropneumothorax are trauma, thoracentesis, surgery, ruptured esophagus and empyema.

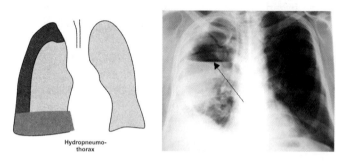

Hydropneumo-
thorax

FIGURE 1.60: CXR showing right hydropneumothorax, note the air-fluid level

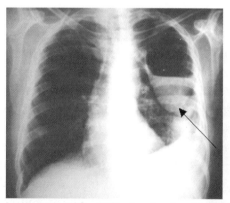

FIGURE 1.61: CXR showing loculated left hydropneumothorax

Tension pneumothorax: It is a life-threatening complication. This leads to a build-up of air increasing intrathoracic pressure and eventually a positive pressure (tension pneumothorax) builds-up. The pressure build-up is large enough to collapse the lung and shift the mediastinum away from the pneumothorax. If it continues, it can compromise venous filling of the heart and even death.

A chest radiograph shows: (1) transradiant hemithorax, (2) mediastinal shift to opposite side, (3) ipsilateral diaphragm depression, and (4) collapse of ipsilateral lung.

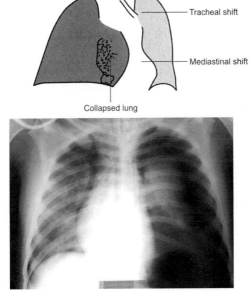

FIGURES 1.62A and B: CXR showing bilateral pneumothorax with shift of mediastinum to the right

Other Complications

Hemothorax: Associated with traumatic pneumothorax. Small amount of serous fluid or blood may accumulate. Blood may clot in pleral space and mimic a mass—fibrin body.

Pyopneumothorax is seen following necrotizing pneumonia or esophageal rupture.

CAUSES OF PNEUMOTHORAX

Spontaneous

Primary	
Secondary	
Airflow obstruction	Asthma, COPD, Cystic fibrosis
Pulmonary infection	Cavitary pneumonia, Tuberculosis, Fungal disease, AIDS, Pneumatocele
Pulmonary infarction	
Neoplasm	Metastatic sarcoma
Diffuse lung disease	Histiocytosis X, Lymphangioleiomyomatosis, Fibrosing alveolitis, other diffuse fibroses
Heritable disorders	Marfan's syndrome
Endometriosis (catamenial pneumothorax)	

Traumatic

Non-iatrogenic	Ruptured esophagus/trachea, Closed chest trauma (+/- rib fracture), Penetrating chest trauma
Iatrogenic	Thoracotomy/thoracocentesis, Percutaneous biopsy, Tracheostomy, Central venous catheterization

Unilateral Hyperlucent Lung

- Chest wall deficiency
  - Poland's syndrome
  - Mastectomy obstructive emphysema

- Mac Leod's syndrome
- Congenital absence of pulmonary artery
- Pulmonary thromboembolism
- Unilateral bullous emphysema
- Lobar collapse
- Pneumothorax
- Technical factors—rotated patient

Pleural Calcification

Pleural calcification is commonly seen in asbestos exposure, empyema, tuberculosis, hemothorax. In empyema the pleural calcifications are irregular and sheet like with pleural thickening. It involves both parietal and visceral pleura. On en face images, they are seen as hazy veil-like dense opacities. In asbestos related pathology, the pleural calcifications are bilateral and discrete collections within the plaques. Usually involves parietal pleura.

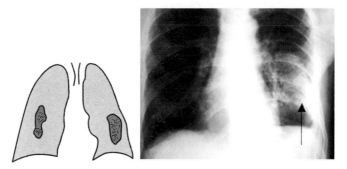

FIGURES 1.63A and B: CXR showing confluent calcification of the left pleura

Pleural Thickening

Pleural thickening can be localized or diffuse.

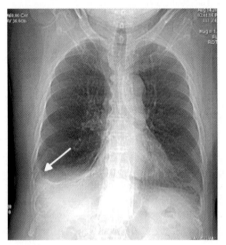

FIGURE 1.64: CXR showing right basal pleural thickening

Causes of Pleural Thickening

- Asbestos; talcosis
- Lung cancer (esp. Pancoast tumor) mesothelioma
- Metastatic disease
- Pleural effusion loculated
- Empyema (pyothorax)
- Old pleuritis, incl. TB
- Old trauma/surgery/hemothorax
- Fungus (histoplasmosis)
- Sarcoidosis
- Parasites

Radiologically, pleural thickening produces soft tissue density shadowing, commonly seen in the dependant parts of the pleural cavity. Blunting of costophrenic angles is the common finding.

Apical pleural cap: These are pleural-based peripheral soft tissue opacities at the lung apex. They can be unilateral/ bilateral. Usually seen in the elderly. Closest differential diagnosis is Pancoast's tumor.

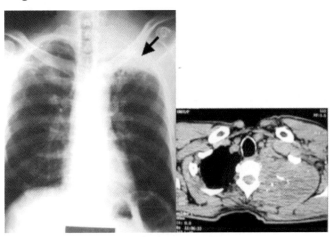

FIGURES 1.65A and B: CXR showing left upper apical opacity caused by Pancoasts tumor

Asbestos-related pleural plaque: These are well-defined soft tissue sheets originating from parietal pleura. They are usually bilateral and situated in the middle and lower zones and over the diaphragm. They usually calcify and give produce a "holly leaf" appearance with sharp angulated edges. Tangential views are helpful in diagnosing pleural plaques. Diffuse pleural thickening is less commonly seen than pleural plaques.

Pleural Thickening with Calcification

- Calcific fibrothorax, i.e. old hemothorax, old pyo-thorax/tuberculous pleurisy
- Asbestos-related pleural disease
- Talc (pleurodesis)
- Rare:
  - Granulomatous infection (histoplasmosis)
  - Calcifying metastases (nodules, not thickening)
  - Calcifying parasitic disease

Pleural Mass Lesions

Pleural-based Mass

- Lung cancer (likelihood depends on age and other risk factors)
- Focal infection/inflammation that is pleural-based
- Metastasis
- Benign spindle-cell tumor (lipoma, neurogenic tumor)
- Fibrous tumor of the pleura ("benign" mesothelioma)
- Loculated effusion/empyema
- Large (raised) pleural plaque
- Chest wall entities
  - Remnants of old chest wall trauma
  - Chest wall tumor: Askin tumor; sarcoma (osteo-sarcoma; chondrosarcoma). Benign: aneurismal bone cyst of rib.

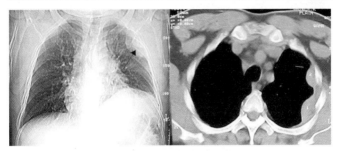

FIGURES 1.66A and B: CXR showing left upper zone pleural opacity, axial CT sections showing nodular pleural thickening

Broad-based Pleural Opacity (Thickening)

- Mesothelioma
- Metastasis
- Benign spindle-cell tumor (lipoma, neurogenic tumor)
- Loculated effusion/empyema
- Fibrothorax/Chronic severe pleural thickening (post-inflammatory)
- Remnants of old chest wall trauma/old hematoma
- Postoperative changes, including flaps.
- Chest wall tumor: Askin tumor; sarcoma (osteosarcoma; chondrosarcoma)
- Large/thick pleural plaque
- Fibrous tumor of the pleura ("benign" mesothelioma)—more often mass-like than plaque-like.

Localized fibrous tumor (localized mesothelioma): These lesions are present in the middle age and are usually benign in nature. Few of them are malignant in nature (10%). These lesions have no relation with asbestos

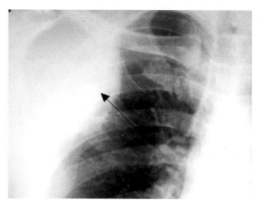

FIGURE 1.67: CXR showing a large pleural-based
opacity on the right upper zone

exposure. Radiologically they appear as solitary pleural
based mass lesion which makes obtuse angle with the chest
wall. It has lobulated margins and sometimes can be
pedunculated. Associated hypertrophic osteoarthropathy
can be present.

DIAPHRAGM

Eventration: It is caused due to absence of a part of
muscle in the diaphragm which is replaced by a thin layer
of connective tissue. It is usually associated with trisomies
13, 18, pulmonary hypoplasia, congenital CMV.
Eventration is more common on the left side.

Radiological features include:
- Hemidiaphragm not visualized
- Multicystic mass in the chest
- Mediastinal shift to opposite side.

Diaphragmatic Hernia

Morgagni Hernia

Hernias through the foramen of Morgagni represent 2–3% of all diaphragmatic hernias. The defect is anterior and retrosternal in location and is usually a right-sided process. The contained contents may include, in order of decreasing frequency, the omentum, colon, stomach, liver, and small intestine. Morgagni hernia can be associated with trauma, severe effort, and obesity. On routine chest radiography, it usually appears as a rounded mass in the right cardiophrenic angle, adjacent to the anterior portion of the chest wall. The differential diagnosis includes pericardial fat pad, pericardial cyst, or solid tumor.

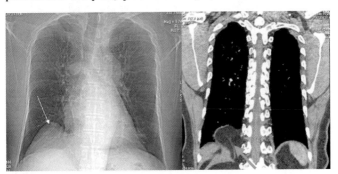

FIGURES 1.68A AND B: Digital scanogram showing right diaphragmatic hump like opacity, coronal reconstructions showing herniation of fat through the diaphragmatic defect

Bochdalek Hernia

Hernias through the foramen of Bochdalek are developmental defects in the posterior part of the diaphragm.

These hernias are usually diagnosed in infants who present with clinical symptoms of pulmonary insufficiency. The herniated contents contain fat and omental tissue in a majority of cases, and also retroperitoneal and intraperitoneal structures can be involved. Left-sided hernias are more common. On conventional radiographs, the hernia may appear as a lung-base soft-tissue-opacity lesion seen posteriorly on lateral images

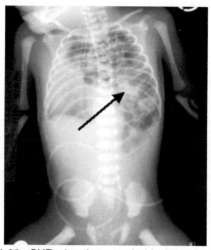

FIGURE 1.69: CXR showing scaphoid abdomen with bowel loops in the left chest causing mediastinal shift

HIATAL HERNIA

Hiatal hernias may be ***sliding or paraesophageal***(less common). Sliding hernias involve upward displacement of the esophageal junction through the esophageal hiatus in the diaphragm into the posterior mediastinum.

Paraesophageal hernias involve protrusion of the stomach into the thorax through the esophageal hiatus. On chest radiographs, a paraesophageal hernia may appear as a soft-tissue-opacity lesion posterior to the heart near the esophageal hiatus.

DIAPHRAGMATIC INJURY

Diaphragmatic injuries occur in 0. 8–8% of patients after blunt trauma. Diaphragmatic injuries remain a diagnostic challenge for both radiologists and surgeons. In most cases, the diagnosis may be obvious at chest radiography and computed tomography (CT); however, some specific signs require careful analysis with CT and magnetic resonance (MR) imaging.

Injuries to the left hemidiaphragm occur three times more frequently than injuries to the right side following blunt trauma, possibly due to a buffering effect of the liver on the right hemidiaphragm Both bilateral tears and extension of tears into the central tendon are uncommon. Mechanisms of injuries include a lateral impact, which distorts the chest wall and shears the diaphragm, and a direct frontal impact, which leads to increased intra-abdominal pressure. Most ruptures are longer than 10 cm and occur at the posterolateral aspect of the hemidiaphragm between the lumbar and intercostal attachments. This is the weakest point of the diaphragm, where the pleuroperitoneal membrane finally closes at embryogenesis. Ruptures of the diaphragm can also occur in its central portion and at its costal attachment.

Penetrating injuries produce small diaphragmatic holes, which are often overlooked.

Common associated injuries include pelvic fractures, splenic injuries, and renal injuries. There is also a high frequency of liver injuries. Thoracic injuries such as pneumothoraces/hemothoraces and rib fractures are seen commonly.

Chest radiography remains valuable in the acute phase for the detection of diaphragmatic rupture. Right diaphragmatic injuries are more difficult to detect on radiographs. The liver serves to block herniation of abdominal contents into the lower right side of the chest. Herniation of the liver is often overlooked. Findings of diaphragmatic tears on chest radiographs include the following: (1) intrathoracic herniation of a hollow viscus (stomach, colon, small bowel) with or without focal constriction of the viscus at the site of the tear—***collar sign*** and (2) visualization of a nasogastric tube above the hemidiaphragm on the left side.

Findings suggestive of hemidiaphragmatic rupture include elevation of the hemidiaphragm, distortion or obliteration of the outline of the hemidiaphragm, and contralateral shift of the mediastinum.

Other associated findings related to the trauma such as pleural effusion, pulmonary contusion or laceration, atelectasis, and phrenic nerve palsy can mimic or mask diaphragmatic injury on chest radiographs.

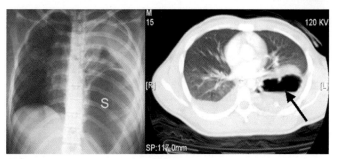

FIGURES 1.70A and B: CXR showing dilated stomach herniating in to left hemithorax follwing a road traffic accident. Axial CT showing the intrathoracic stomach

UNILATERAL ELEVATED HEMIDIAPHRAGM

- ***Causes above the diaphragm:***
  Pulmonary collapse
  Phrenic nerve palsy
  Pulmonary hypoplasia
  Pulmonary thromboembolism
  Pleurisy
- ***Diaphragmatic causes:***
  Eventration
  Trauma
- ***Causes below the diaphragm:***
  Gaseous distension of stomach
  Subphrenic mass/abscess
  Hepatic/splenic abscess
- ***Scoliosis***
- ***Posture*** – lateral decubitus(dependent side)

BILATERAL ELEVATED DIAPHRAGMS

- *Causes above the diaphragms*
  Bilateral pulmonary collapse
  Diffuse pulmonary fibrosis
- *Causes below the diaphragm*
  Ascites
  Pregnancy
  Pneumoperitoneum
  Hepatoslenomegaly
  Large intraabdominal tumor
  Intestinal obstruction
  Post abdominal surgery
- *Diaphragmatic causes:*
  Bilateral diaphragmatic paralysis
- *Poor inspiratory effort*
- *Obesity.*

PNEUMOMEDIASTINUM

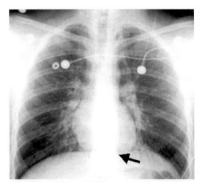

FIGURE 1.71: CXR showing continuous
diaphragm sign of pneumomediastinum

Pneumomediastinum may result from a variety of causes that may be either intrathoracic (e.g. narrowed or plugged airway, straining against a closed glottis, blunt chest trauma, alveolar rupture) or extrathoracic (e.g. sinus fracture, iatrogenic manipulation in dental extraction, perforation of a hollow viscus). The radiographic signs of pneumomediastinum depend on the depiction of normal anatomic structures that are outlined by the air as it leaves the mediastinum. These signs include the thymic sail sign, "ring around the artery" sign, tubular artery sign, double bronchial wall sign, continuous **diaphragm** sign, and extrapleural sign. In distal esophageal rupture, air may migrate from the mediastinum into the pulmonary ligament. Pneumomediastinum may be difficult to differentiate from medial pneumothorax and pneumo-pericardium. Occasionally, normal anatomic structures (eg, major fissure, anterior junction line) may simulate air within the mediastinum.

BASICS OF CARDIAC DIAGNOSIS FROM CHEST X-RAY

THE FIRST OBSERVATION USUALLY MADE IS THAT OF THE HEART SIZE: The cardiothoracic ratio.

Heart Size

The cardiothoracic ratio is the maximum transverse diameter of the heart divided by the greatest internal diameter of the thoracic cage (from inside of rib to inside of rib).

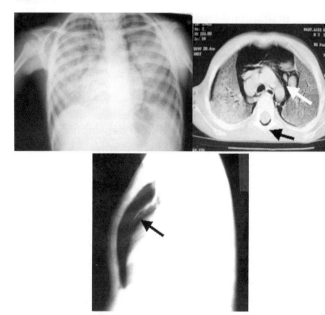

FIGURES 1.72A to C: A) CXR showing bilateral pneumothorax and pneumomediastinum. B) Axial CT section showing pneumomediastinum and pneumorachis. Lungs appear white due acute interstitial pneumonia. C) Lateral X-ray showing increased anterior mediastinal lucency.

In normal people, the cardiothoracic ratio is usually less than 50%. Therefore, the cardiothoracic ratio is a handy way of separating most normal hearts from most abnormal hearts.

But it is not without pitfalls. A heart may be greater than 50% of the cardiothoracic ratio and still be a normal heart.

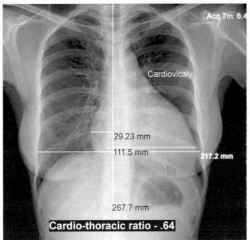

FIGURE 1.73: Method of measuring CTR

This can occur if there is an extracardiac cause of cardiac enlargement. Extracardiac causes of cardiac enlargement include:

Inability to take a deep breath because of

- Obesity
- Pregnancy, or
- Ascites

Or abnormalities of the chest that compress the heart such as

- Pectus excavatum deformity, or
- Straight Back syndrome

Sometimes the heart can be smaller than 50% of the cardiothoracic ratio but still be an abnormal heart. This occurs when there is something obstructing the flow of

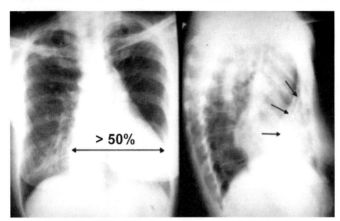

FIGURES 1.74A AND B: Pectus excavatum deformity causing pseudo-cardiomegaly

blood from the ventricles since the ventricles respond at first by undergoing hypertrophy, which does not produce cardiomegaly.

Since not all abnormal hearts are enlarged, definition of cardiac disease in those individuals depends on an assessment of the contours of the heart on the frontal film.

Cardiac Contours

1. On the right side of the heart, the first contour is that of the **ascending aorta**.

This is a low density, almost-straight edge visible just to the right of the trachea anatomically representing the superior vena cava and the brachiocephalic vein but in practice reflecting the size of the ascending aorta. So we shall call this contour the ascending aorta.

The ascending aorta can be small as in ASD or it can be convex outward as in aortic stenosis, aortic regurgitation, and hypertensive cardiovascular disease. The ascending aorta should never project farther to the right than the right heart border in a normal person.

2. Just below the ascending aorta is an indentation where the so-called "**double density of left atrial enlargement**" will appear when the left atrium enlarges toward the right side of the heart.

Normally, the left atrium forms no border of the heart in the frontal projection. When the left atrium enlarges, it may produce two abnormal contours of the heart.

Where the ascending aorta meets the right atrium, there is usually an indentation. In patients with an enlarged left atrium which projects to the right, there will be two overlapping densities seen where this indentation normally is. One of the densities is the normal right atrium. The other overlapping density is the enlarged left atrium.

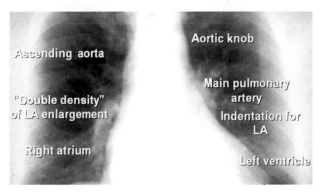

FIGURE 1.75: Normal cardiac contours

The double density may occasionally be seen in normal individuals; always check left heart border for straightening.

3. The last contour on the right side of the heart is the **right atrium**. In an adult, every disease that causes enlargement of the right atrium also produces enlargement of the right ventricle. So we can consider the right atrium and ventricle together as a single functional unit in adults and we will estimate right-sided cardiac enlargement by observing another cardiac contour, but not the right atrium.

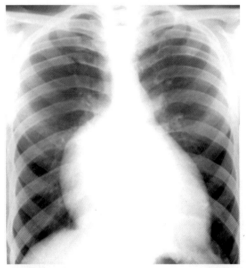

FIGURE 1.76: Enlarged RA seen in Ebsteins

Therefore, for this system the right atrium is not an important contour.

Now we move to the left heart border and start at the top.

4. On the left side of the heart, the first contour is the **aortic knob**. The aortic knob is a radiographic structure that is formed by the foreshortened aortic arch and a portion of the descending aorta.

In normal people the aortic knob measures less than 35 mm when measured from the lateral border of the trachea to the lateral border of the aortic knob.

The knob will be greater than 35 mm due to increased pressure, flow, or changes in the elasticity of the wall e.g. cystic medial necrosis, dissection of the aorta.

5. Just below the aortic knob is the **main or undivided segment of the pulmonary artery**. The main pulmonary is very important in this system and forms the cornerstone for two of the main categories of disease to follow.

First, you must be able to find the main pulmonary artery segment. Then, you can measure it.

You can find the main pulmonary artery by either locating the first contour below the aortic knob or by finding the adjacent squiggly vessels that are the left pulmonary artery. The main and left pulmonary arteries are always adjacent to each other.

We can measure the main pulmonary artery by drawing a tangent line from the apex of the left ventricle to the aortic knob and then measuring along a perpendicular to that tangent line, the distance between the tangent and the main pulmonary artery.

In normal people, the distance between the tangent and the main pulmonary artery lies within a range of values between 0 mm (the main pulmonary is touching the tangent line) to as far away from the tangent line (medially) as 15 mm.

Therefore, this sets up two major categories of abnormality.

First, the main pulmonary artery may project beyond the tangent line (greater than 0 mm).

This can occur if there is increased pressure or increased flow in the pulmonary circuit.

Second, the main pulmonary artery may project more than 15 mm away from the tangent line.

This can occur either because there is something intrinsically wrong with the pulmonary artery such as

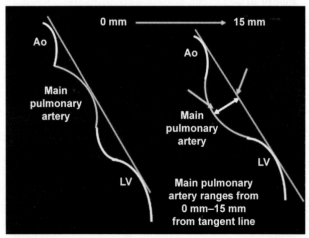

FIGURE 1.77: Schematic showing the MPA measurement

absence or hypoplasia of the pulmonary artery, e.g. Tetralogy of Fallot, truncus. But, these diseases are uncommon in adults.

The other reason the main pulmonary artery may be more than 15 mm from the tangent line is the left ventricle and/or aortic knob may enlarge and push the tangent line away from pulmonary artery, e.g. atherosclerosis. These are very common diseases.

Young females may normally have prominence of the MPA but rarely does the main pulmonary artery project beyond the tangent.

6. Just below the main pulmonary artery segment (area between the main pulmonary artery and the left ventricle) is a little concavity where the left atrium, when it enlarges on the left side of the heart, will appear.

Filling in at this concavity by an enlarged left atrium produces "straightening" of the left heart border. It may be seen in mitral disease or shunt (VSD, PDA) and rarely left atrial myxoma, papillary muscle dysfunction and chronic CHF.

Sometimes, the left atrial appendage may enlarge as well. A convexity at this contour means the left atrial appendage is enlarged and is seen in mitral valvular disease, usually mitral stenosis.

7. The last cardiac contour is the **left ventricle**.

The best way to evaluate which ventricle is enlarged (i.e. right or left) is to look at the corresponding outflow tracts for each ventricle.

If the heart is enlarged and the main pulmonary artery is large (sticks out beyond the tangent line), then the cardiomegaly is made up of at least right ventricular enlargement.

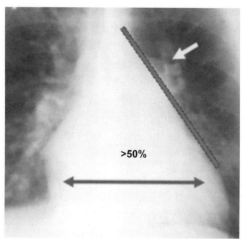

FIGURE 1.78: X-ray showing cardiomegaly with enlarged MPA suggesting RV enlargement as a cause for cardiomegaly

If the heart is enlarged and the aorta is prominent (ascending, knob, descending), then the cardiomegaly is made up of at least left ventricular enlargement

Once one ventricle is determined to be enlarged, then the other ventricle may also be enlarged but there is no way to identify this with a chest X-ray.

Pulmonary Vasculature

It is important to know that the pulmonary vasculature will fall into one of the following four categories:

1. Normal
2. Pulmonary venous hypertension
3. Pulmonary arterial hypertension
4. Increased flow

1. Measure the right descending pulmonary artery (RDPA).

The RDPA is visible on almost all chest films as a large vessel just to the right of the right heart border. Its diameter can be measured at about the level of the indentation between the ascending aorta and the right atrium.

In normal people, **the right descending pulmonary artery is less the 17 mm in diameter**.

2. Evaluate the distribution of flow from apex to base

In normal people, in the erect position, the blood flow to the bases is greater than the blood flow to the apices. This is due to the effect of gravity. In normal people, the size of the vessels at the base will therefore be greater than the size of the vessels at the apex.

In people with **pulmonary venous hypertension**, the blood flow to the apex becomes equal to or greater than the blood flow to the base. Therefore the size of the vessels at the apex becomes equal to or greater than the size of the vessels at the bases – a reversal of the normal distribution pattern. This is known as **cephalization**.

3. Evaluate the distribution of flow from central to peripheral

Normally, the pulmonary vessels taper gradually from central to peripheral. It doesn't matter whether they are arteries or veins and it doesn't matter whether it is the lung or any other organ, blood vessels taper gradually from central to peripheral.

In **pulmonary arterial hypertension**, there is a redistribution of flow in the lungs from central to peripheral such that the peripheral vessels appear too small for the size of the central vessels from which they come. This discrepancy in the size of the central pulmonary vessels (which are large) compared to the peripheral pulmonary vasculature (which even though it is small is still indistinguishable from normal) is called **pruning**.

Using the size of the RDPA and the distribution of flow in the lungs—apex to base and central to peripheral, we can define the four states of the pulmonary vasculature.

In NORMAL PULMONARY VASCULATURE

The right descending pulmonary artery is less than 17mm

The lower lobe vessels are larger than the upper lobe vessels.

There is a gradual tapering of the blood vessels from central to peripheral.

In PULMONARY VENOUS HYPERTENSION

The right descending pulmonary artery is usually greater than 17 mm.

The upper lobe vessels are equal to or greater than the size of the lower lobe vessels (cephalization).

There is a gradual tapering of the blood vessels from central to peripheral.

In **PULMONARY ARTERIAL HYPERTENSION**

The right descending pulmonary artery is greater than 17 mm.

The lower lobe vessels are larger than the upper lobe vessels.

There is a rapid decrease in the size of the peripheral vessels relative to the central vessels from which they come (pruning).

In **INCREASED FLOW**

The right descending pulmonary artery is greater than 17 mm.

The lower lobe vessels are larger than the upper lobe vessels.

There is a gradual tapering of the blood vessels from central to peripheral.

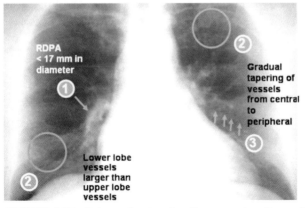

FIGURE 1.79: Schematic showing the normal pattern of pulmonary vessels

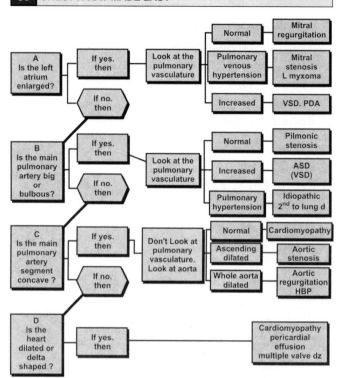

FIGURE 1.80: Flow chart showing a basic classroom approach

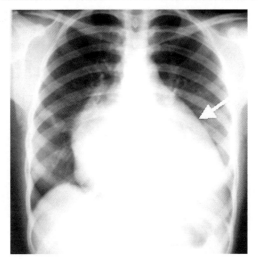

FIGURE 1.81: CXR showing straightening of left cardiac border

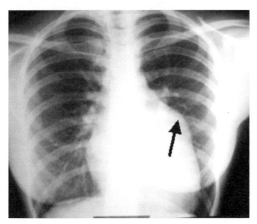

FIGURE 1.82: CXR showing enlarged left pulmonary artery

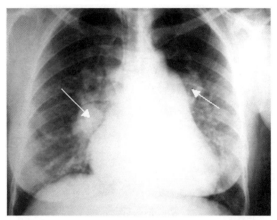

FIGURE 1.83: CXR showing enlargement of RPDA and left pulmonary artery

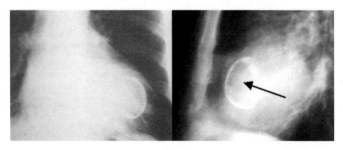

FIGURE 1.84: CXR showing left apical arc like calcification of the left ventricular aneurysm

PLAIN FILM APPROACH TO CRITICAL CARE PATIENT
WITH CXR FINDINGS OF PULMONARY CONGESTION

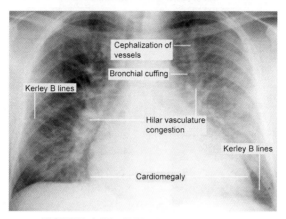

FIGURE 1.85: CXR showing classical features of pulmonary edema

Table 1.1: Differential diagnosis of different causes of pulmonary edema

Radiological sign	Cardiogenic	Renal	Capillary injury
Heart shape	L-sided enlargement	R&L enlargement	Normal
Vascular pedicle width (SV)	+	++	Normal
Pulmonary blood distribution	Balanced or inverted	Balanced	Normal
Pulmonary blood volume	Normal or +	++	Normal
Septal lines	++	+	No
Peribronchial & vessel cuffing	+	+	No
Air Bronchogram	+	+	++
Lung opacity distribution	Central and peripheral	Central	Peripheral & central
Pleural effusion	++	+	Uncommon
Soft-tissue chest wall	+	++	Normal

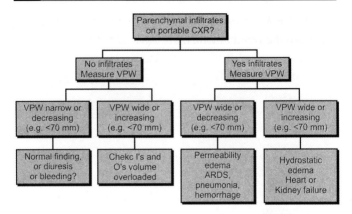

FIGURE 1.86: Use of the vascular pedicle width from portable supine CXR

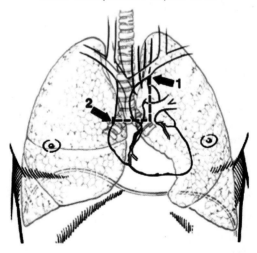

FIGURE 1.87: Schematic showing the site of measuring the vascular pedicle. Normal VPW range is 48 ± 5 mm

The VPW is measured by (1) dropping a perpendicular line from the point at which the left subclavian artery exits the aortic arch and (2) measuring across to the point at which the superior vena cava crosses the right mainstem bronchus.

Pericardial Effusion

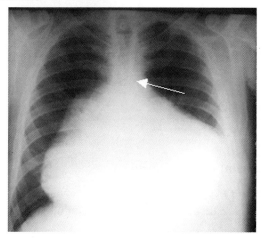

FIGURE 1.88: CXR showing the classical appearance of enlarged heart with a narrow pedicle

X-Ray Signs of Pericardial Effusion

- Distinctness of the epicardial fat planes
- Normal pulmonary vasculature despite cardiomegaly
- Obliteration of reterosternal space
- Water bottle appearance of the enlarged cardiac silhouette
- Bilateral hilar overlay.

Pericardial Calcifications

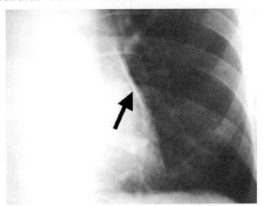

FIGURE 1.89: CXR showing linear
pericardial calcification

Pericardial Calcification

- It is a consequence of tissue injury from inflammation,
  trauma causes include viral, tuberculosis, pyogenic
  infection
- Incidence in patients with constructive pericarditis is
  50 to 70%
- The atrioventricular, interventricular groove and
  diaphragmatic border of the heart are common sites
  for calcification
- The left atrium and left ventricle are usually spared.

CHAPTER 2

Disease Pattern

- The chest radiograph is a composite image of the thoracic anatomy depicted in a gray scale based on the electron densities of the thoracic contents.
- The conspicuity of a region of interest is dependent on:
  - The region's attenuation of the X-ray beam
  - The additive attenuations of all structures anterior and posterior to it
  - The contrast between it, and its surrounding structures.

Opacities can be classified as:
- An opacity significantly denser than the heart.
  - Calcium
  - Metal
  - Bone
- An opacity equivalent or slightly denser than the heart
  - Water
  - Cells
  - Hemorrhage
- An opacity not as dense as the heart-Hazy
  - Fat
  - Water
  - Cells
  - Hemorrhage

Other Descriptions

- Shape
  - Linear
  - Tubular
  - Round

- Boarders
  - Smooth
  - Irregular/Shaggy

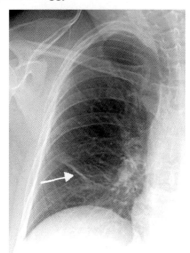

FIGURE 2.1: A shadow resembling a line; hence, any elongated opacity of approximately uniform width-linear atelectasis

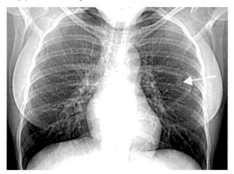

FIGURE 2.2: Tubular opacity— pulmonary AVM

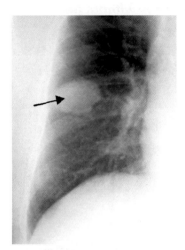

FIGURE 2.3: Round opacity—
pulmonary mass

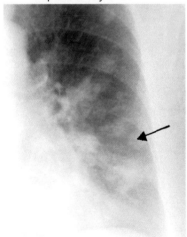

FIGURE 2.4: Irregular opacity—metastasis

Localized Opacity without Segmental Distribution

Opacity with a uniform (homogenous) density
Uni-/bilateral
Focal rather than diffuse
Air bronchogram is almost invariably present and should not be misinterpreted as e/o inhomogeneity.

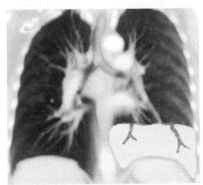

FIGURE 2.5

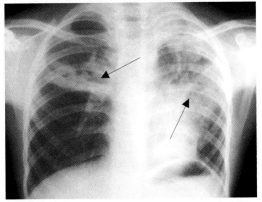

FIGURE 2.6: CXR showing bilateral opacities with air bronchograms

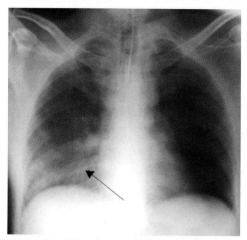

FIGURE 2.7: CXR showing right lower lobe opacity

Diffuse Disease with a Predominantly Reticular Pattern (See Fig. 2.9)

Thin linear opacities having a net-like appearance.

Opacities may be diffuse involving all lobes of both lungs, although they are often most marked in some regions.

The pattern may be related to such pathologic abnormalities as thickened interlobular septa, parenchymal cystic spaces, or interstitial fibrosis ("honeycombing").

Diffuse Disease with a Predominantly Military Nodular Pattern (See Figs 2.10 and 2.11)

Diffuse nodular opacities typically measuring less than 5 mm in diameter.

The nodules may have well or poorly defined margins.

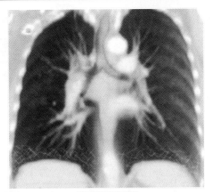

FIGURE 2.8

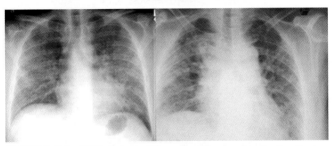

FIGURE 2.9: CXR in two different patients classical reticular opacities

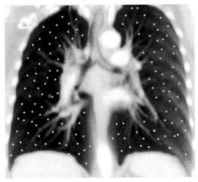

FIGURE 2.10

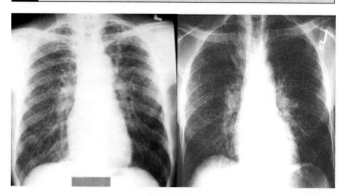

FIGURE 2.11: CXR showing classical miliary modular pattern

Generalized Pulmonary Translucency

Diffuse hyperlucency of the lungs associated with a splaying of the pulmonary vascular bundle.

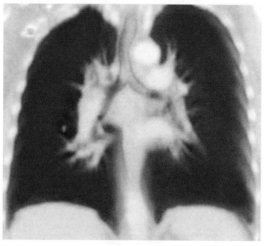

FIGURE 2.12

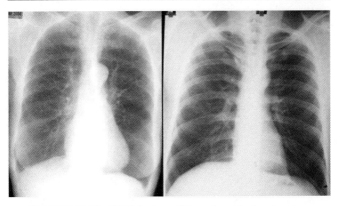

FIGURE 2.13: CXR in two different patients showing features of hyperinflation

Unilateral, Lobar, or Segmental Pulmonary Hyperlucency

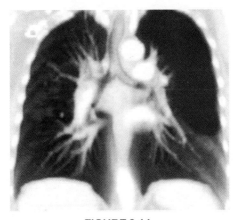

FIGURE 2.14

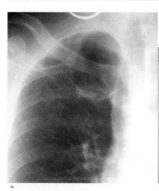
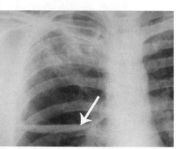

FIGURE 2.15 A and B: CXR showing right upper lobe bulla in two different patients. In Fig B note the air fluid level indicating infection (arrow)

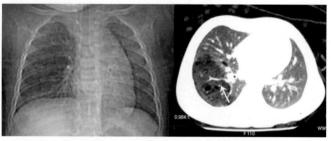

FIGURE 2.16: Digital scanogram and axial HRCT showing a right lower lobe lucency with multiple cysts suggestive of congenital cystadenamatoid malformation (arrow)

Hilar and Mediastinal Lymph Node Enlargement

Expanded often lobulated hilar region.
Uni-/bilateral

Mediastinal disease most often manifested as enlargement of right paratracheal, subcarinal, aortopulmonary or paraspinal lymph nodes.

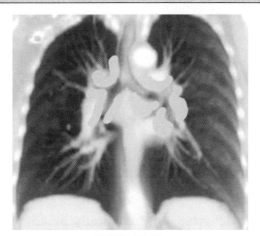

FIGURE 2.17

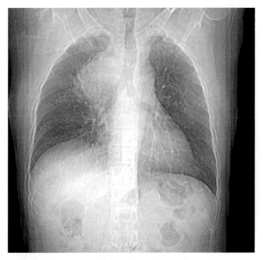

FIGURE 2.18: CXR showing a large right
paratracheal node

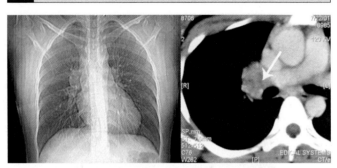

FIGURE 2.19: Digital scanogram and axial CECT showing right hilar node (arrow)

Masses Situated Predominantly in Anterior Mediastinal Compartment

Anterior mediastinum is bounded.

Anteriorly by the sternum.

Posteriorly by the pericardium, aorta, and brachio-cephalic vessels.

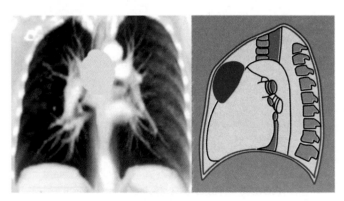

FIGURE 2.20

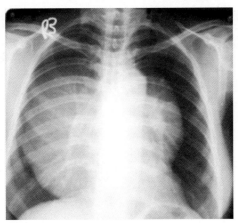

FIGURE 2.21: CXR showing large well marginated opacity through which the right hilum is well seen (case of anterior mediastinal cyst)

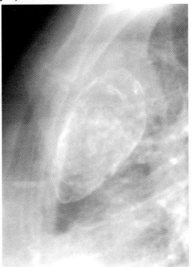

FIGURE 2.22: Lateral X-ray showing a well marginated calcified mass in the anterior mediastinum

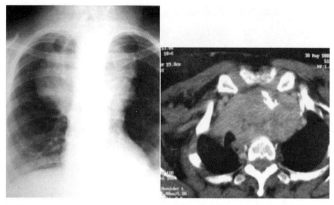

FIGURE 2.23: CXR and axial CT section showing a large heterogenous mass in the superior and anterior mediastinum —case of large retrosternal goitre

For practical reasons, a mass is considered to lie in the anterior compartment when it is situated in the region anterior to a line drawn along the anterior border of the trachea and the posterior border of the heart.

Masses Situated Predominantly in Middle and Posterior Mediastinal Compartments

Middle mediastinum contains → heart, major vessels, trachea and main bronchi, lymph nodes, phrenic and vagus nerves.

Posterior mediastinum contains → descending thoracic aorta, esophagus, thoracic duct, vagus nerves and lymph nodes.

On lateral CXR, these 2 compartments are considered together.

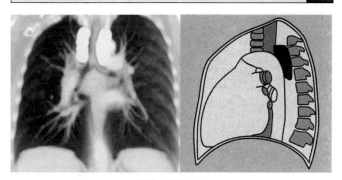

FIGURE 2.24

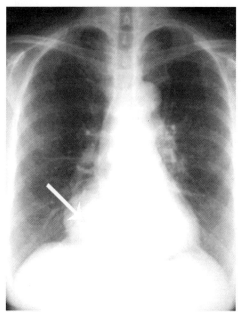

FIGURE 2.25 CXR showing a right cardiophrenic angle opacity—case of pericardial cyst (arrow)

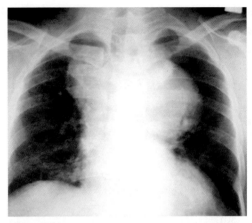

FIGURE 2.26: CXR showing a lobulated opacity (arrow) causing widening of mediastinum—case of aortic arch aneurysm

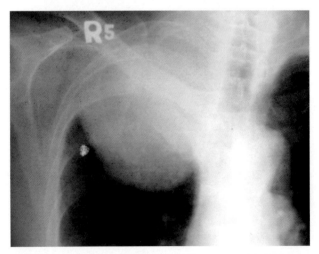

FIGURE 2.27: CXR showing a well marginated right upper zone opacity (case of neural tumour)

- Lesion can be considered to lie in the middle or posterior compartment when it is located below a line drawn through anterior aspect of trachea and posterior aspect of heart and the line drawn through the anterior margins of vertebral bodies.

Masses Situated in the Paravertebral Region

Posterior limit of mediastinum is formed by the anterior surface of the vertebral column.

On lateral CXR, a mass can be considered to be in the paravertebral region when it lies posterior to the anterior surface of vertebral bodies.

Localized Pleural Based/Chest Wall Opacity (See Figs 2.29 and 2.30)

Peripheral mass with obtuse margins that abuts the chest wall and pleura with or without rib destruction.

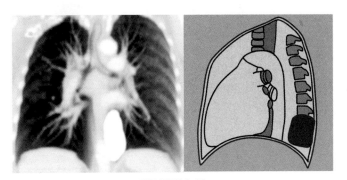

FIGURE 2.28

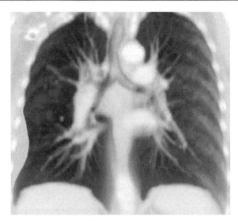

FIGURE 2.29

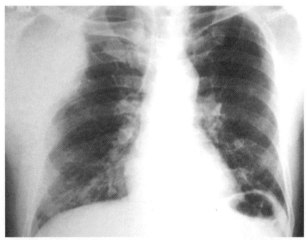

FIGURE 2.30: CXR showing right upper zone pleural based soft tissue mass

Diffuse Pleural Thickening

Diffuse in this context is defined as an uninterrupted pleural opacity extending over at least 1/4th of the chest wall with or without obliteration of the costophrenic sulcus.

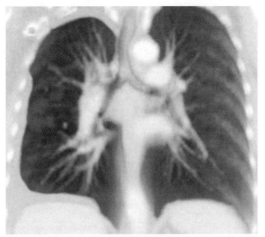

FIGURE 2.31

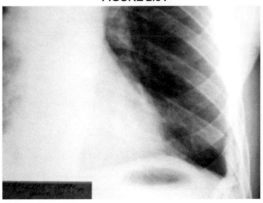

FIGURE 2.32: CXR showing left lateral and basal pleural thickening

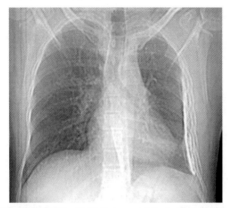

FIGURE 2.33: Digital scanogram showing left pleural diffuse thickening with calcification

Pleural Effusion with Large Cardiac Silhouette

Enlargement of the cardiac silhouette is considered to be present when an increase in its size is demonstrated on serial radiographs or the cardiac silhouette:thorax ratio is greater than 1:2 (50%).

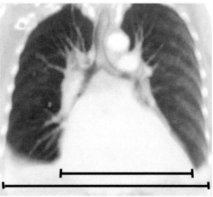

FIGURE 2.34

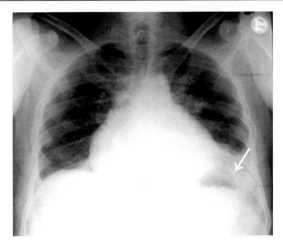

FIGURE 2.35: CXR showing enlarged heart with bilateral pleural effusion more evident on the left side

Pleural Effusion without Pulmonary Disease

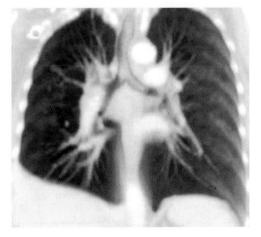

FIGURE 2.36

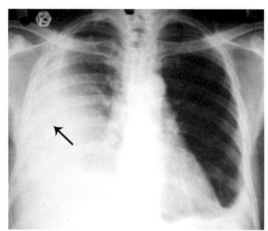

FIGURE 2.37: CXR showing bilateral pleural effusion more evident on the right side

Pleural Effusion with Pulmonary Disease

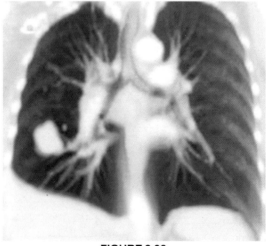

FIGURE 2.38

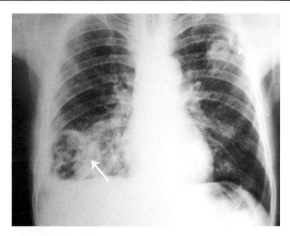

FIGURE 2.39: CXR showing right lower zone pneumonitis with pleural effusion. Note the left upper lobe fungal ball

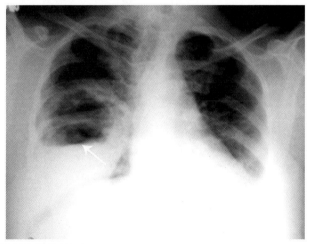

FIGURE 2.40: CXR showing right lower lobe abscess with pleural effusion. Note the air fluid level (arrow)

Localized Opacity with Segmental Distribution

An opacity with a uniform (homogeneous) density located in the site of one or more bronchopulmonary segments. Masses of infective pneumonia can cause this appearance.

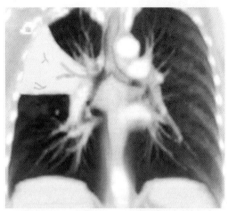

FIGURE 2.41

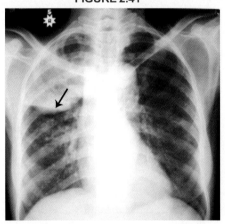

FIGURE 2.42: CXR showing right upper lobe mass causing fissural bulging (arrow)

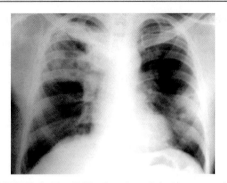

FIGURE 2.43: CXR showing right upper and left lobe consolidations

Cystic and Cavitary Disease

This pattern includes all forms of pulmonary disease characterized by one or several circumscribed air-containing spaces, each of which is bordered by distinct walls, including cavitated pneumonia or carcinoma, and cystic bronchiectasis.

An air-fluid level may or may not be present.

Cavities may be single or multiple.

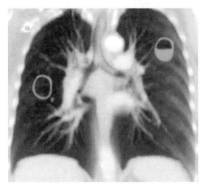

FIGURE 2.44

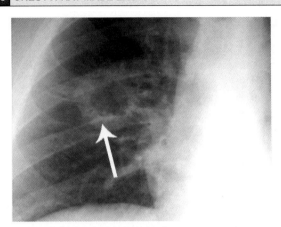

FIGURE 2.45: CXR showing right mid zone thick walled cavity with adjacent satellite lesions abscess

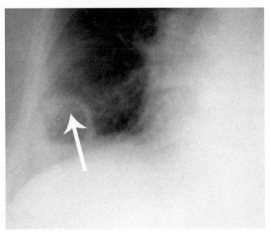

FIGURE 2.46: CXR showing right lower zone costophrenic angle cavity with fluid level (arrow)

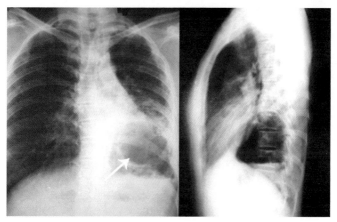

FIGURE 2.47: CXR PA and lateral view showing a large cyst with air fluid level and uniform thick walls

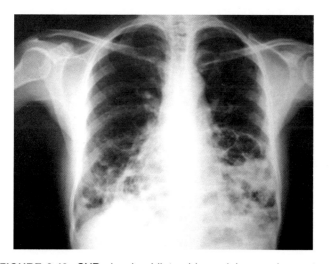

FIGURE 2.48: CXR showing bilateral lower lobe conglomerate cyst with few cysts showing fluid levels—case of infected bronchiectasis

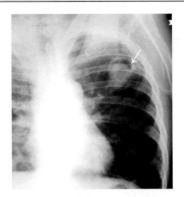

FIGURE 2.49: Left upper lobe cavity with fungal ball—classical case of air crescent sign of fungal ball

Solitary Pulmonary Mass

A discrete opacity >3 cm in diameter.

It may have any contour (smooth, lobulated, or umbilicated) May or may not be calcified.

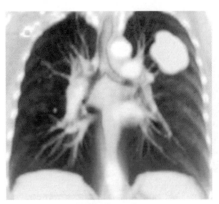

FIGURE 2.50

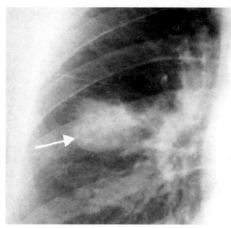

FIGURE 2.51: CXR showing right mid zone opacity

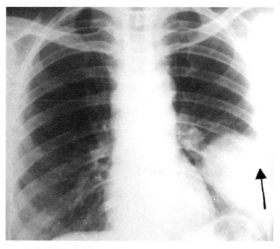

FIGURE 2.52: CXR showing left lower lobe
soft tissue opacity

Multiple Pulmonary Nodules or Masses, with or Without Cavitation

- Multiple opacities > 5 mm in diameter.
- They may have any contour (smooth, lobulated, or umbilicated).
- May or may not be calcified.

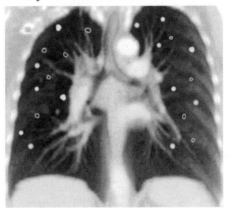

FIGURE 2.53

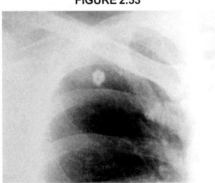

FIGURE 2.54: CXR showing right upper lobe calcified nodule

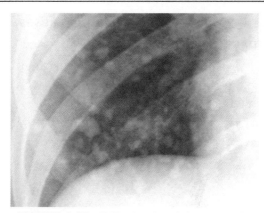

FIGURE 2.55: CXR showing right mid and lower zone multiple calcified nodules

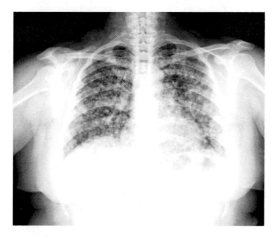

FIGURE 2.56: CXR showing bilateral multiple lung nodules—Typical features of metastasis

Diffuse Disease with a Predominantly Air-Space Pattern

Opacities involving several lobes of both lungs.
Though the disease is widespread, it does not necessarily affect all lung regions uniformly.

For example, lower lung zones may be involved to a greater or lesser degree than the upper.

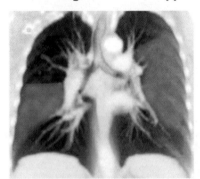

FIGURE 2.57

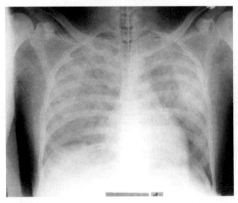

FIGURE 2.58: ARDS CXR in a patient with history of toxic gas inhalation showing bilateral diffuse parenchymal opacities

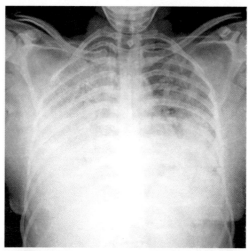

FIGURE 2.59: CXR showing diffuse parenchymal opacity in a patient with acute interstitial pneumonia

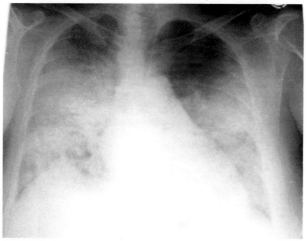

FIGURE 2.60: Pulmonary edema with classical batswing appearance

FIBROCAVITARY DISEASE

Patterns of Tuberculosis

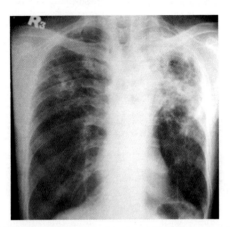

FIGURE 2.61: CXR showing bilateral upper lobe fibrocavitary disease, more evident on the left side

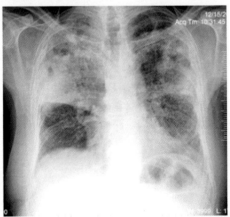

FIGURE 2.62: CXR showing bilateral upper lobe cavitary consolidation

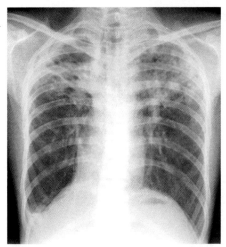

FIGURE 2.63: CXR showing bilateral upper lobe fibrosis with sequelae

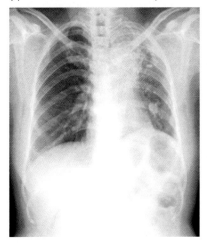

FIGURE 2.64: CXR showing left upper lobe fibrosis with collapse. Note the elevated left hemidiaphragm

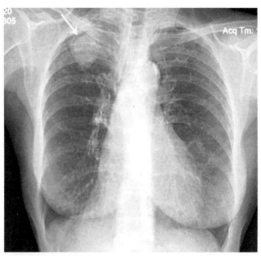

FIGURE 2.65: CXR showing right upper lobe cavity with fungal ball. Note the Monacls sign (air crescent).

CHAPTER 3

Differential Diagnosis

Normal CXR

1. Cardiac diameter < ½ thoracic width-measured inside ribs
   - PA, inspiratory, erect film
2. ~ 1.5 cm change in diameter between inspiration/expiration
3. Right heart border
   i. SVC ± azygous vein
   ii. Right PA
   iii. RA ± LA
4. Left heart border
   i. Aortic arch
   ii. PA/aortic angle
   iii. Left PA
   iv. LA appendage
   v. Left ventricle

"Apparently" Normal CXR

1. Breast shadows ? mastectomy
2. Superior mediastinal masses
3. Posterior mediastinal masses-look behind the heart
4. Ribs-notching, tumors, cervical ribs.
5. Bones-clavicles and hyperparathyroidism
   - Spine
6. Labels-dextrocardia
7. Beneath diaphragm-gas,
8. Lungs-small pneumothorax
   - Apical lung disease

Respiratory Distress and "Normal" CXR

1. Pulmonary embolism
2. Asthma
3. Airway obstruction-FB, secretions, ETT cuff, epiglottis, croup, etc.

COIN LESION ON CXR

Single—Common;
1. 1° carcinoma
2. Metastasis
3. Hamartoma
4. Granuloma
5. Tuberculosis

Multiple—Common
1. Metastases
2. Granulomata
3. Abscesses
4. Septic emboli
5. Multiple pulmonary emboli
6. Hydatid

Single—Uncommon;
1. Hydatid
2. AV malformation
3. Abscess
4. Pulmonary embolus/infarction
5. Adenoma
6. Hematoma

7. Bronchogenic cyst
8. Wegener's granulomata
9. Progressive massive thrombosis

Multiple—Common
1. AV malformation
2. Lymphoma
3. Wegener's granulomatosis
4. Rheumatoid lung

Features suggestive of ***malignancy***,
1. Male > female
2. Smoker
3. Age > 70 yrs ~ 50 %
   50-70 yrs ~ 25%
   < 35 yrs < 1%
4. Increase size < 2 yrs
5. Absence of calcification

Lobar Consolidation

CXR Appearances
1. Homogeneous opacity
2. **No** "air" bronchogram
3. Structural displacement
   - Fissures
   - Vessels
   - Mediastinum, trachea
4. Elevation of hemidiaphragm
5. Compensatory expansion

Lobar Pneumonia

1. Homogeneous opacity
2. "Air" bronchogram
3. No structural displacement
   Klebsiella → bulging fissures
4. "Paralysis" of hemidiaphragm
5. ± pleural effusion, cavitation

Common Causes

1. Sputum retention
2. Malposition of ETT
3. Mechanical ventilation
4. Postoperative-CABG
   - Upper GIT
5. Carcinoma, adenoma
6. Foreign body

Bronchopneumonia

1. Patchy basal opacities
2. "Air" bronchogram
3. Clinical signs over affected area

Butterfly Appearance

1. Pulmonary edema
   i. Cardiogenic
   ii. Non-cardiogenic
2. Pneumonia
3. Alveolar proteinosis
4. Lymphoma

Reversed Butterfly Appearance

1. Pulmonary eosinophilia
2. Sarcoidosis

Bilateral Hilar Enlargement

1. ***Lymphadenopathy***
   i. Lymphatic leukemia
   ii. Lymphoma
   iii. Hodgkin's disease
   iv. Carcinoma-renal cell
      - Melanoma
      - Head/neck carcinoma
   v. Sarcoidosis
   vi. Infectious mononucleosis
   vii. Whooping cough
   viii. Primary tuberculosis-rarely, usually unilateral

2. ***Vascular***
   i. Pulmonary hypertension- chronic lung disease
      - Multiple pulmonary emboli
      - Primary pulmonary hypertension
   ii. L→ R shunts-ASD, VSD
   iii. Pulmonary artery dilatation
       Post-pulmonary stenosis
       Congenital large pulmonary artery
       Aneurysm

Cavitating Lesion on CXR

1. Common
    i. Carcinoma
    ii. Infection-TB, abscess, hydatid
    iii. Pulmonary emboli, infarct
    iv. Septic emboli, infarct
2. Uncommon
    i. Lymphoma
    ii. Hematoma
    iii. Bulla
    iv. Pneumatocele
    v. Wegener's
    vi. Bronchogenic cyst

Lung Infections

1. Lobar/segmental—bacterial, atypical
2. Expanding lobar—Staph., gram-negatives, *Klebsiella*, anaerobes
3. Cavitating—Staph., gram-negatives, *Klebsiella*, anaerobes, fungi
4. Generalized alveolar—bacterial, pneumocystis
5. Generalized interstitial—viral, TB, atypical, fungal, pneumocystis
6. Crescentic—hydatid, fungal
7. Effusion—bacterial, TB
8. Extrapulmonary—actinomycosis, hydatid
9. Pneumothorax—Staph., *Klebsiella*
10. Lymphadenopathy—viral, TB, fungal, actinomycosis

Apical Disease on CXR

1. TB
2. Other infections
3. Bronchogenic carcinoma—Pancoast's tumor
4. Metastases
5. Pleural thickening
6. Extra-pleural disease

Peribronchial Thickening

1. Chronic bronchitis
2. Asthma
3. Edema
4. Bronchiectasis
5. Cystic fibrosis

Diffuse Pulmonary Infiltrates

NB: Divide into *acute* or *chronic*

1. *Acute*
    i. Cardiogenic edema-LVF, MS
    ii. ARDS-sepsis, trauma, transfusion reaction, fat emboli, etc.
    iii. Infection-bacterial, viral, fungal, protozoal
    iv. Hemorrhage-contusions, trauma
        - infarction, Goodpasture's, coagulopathy
        - idiopathic hemosiderosis
    v. Aspiration
    vi. Pulmonary eosinophilia

NB: in severe COAD the distribution of edema is *patchy*

2. **Subacute** → above plus,
    i. Alveolar proteinosis
   ii. Lymphangitis carcinomatosis
  iii. Malignancy-lymphoma, alveolar cell carcinoma
   iv. Sarcoidosis

3. **Chronic: upper zones**
    i. Aspergillosis
   ii. Ankylosing spondylitis, ulcerative colitis
  iii. Extrinsic fibrosing alveolitis-organic dust inhalation
   iv. Silicosis
    v. Sarcoidosis
   vi. Tuberculosis
  vii. Rare-radiotherapy, histiocytosis X

4. **Chronic: lower zones**
    i. Asbestosis
   ii. Aspiration-chronic, recurrent
  iii. Intrinsic fibrosing alveolitis-RA, SLE, scleroderma, drugs, etc.
   iv. Bronchiectasis
    v. Chronic bronchitis, COAD
   vi. Pulmonary eosinophilia-protozoal, drugs
  vii. Rare von Recklinghausen's
 viii. Drugs
       Amiodarone, bleomycin, busulphan, methysergide, hydrallazine, procainamide, sulphonamides

Upper Lobe

1. S-silicosis (progressive massive fibrosis)
   - Sarcoidosis

2. C-coal workers pneumoconiosis
3. H-histiocytosis X
4. A-ankylosing spondylitis, aspergillosis
5. R-radiation
6. T-TB

Lower Lobe

1. R-rheumatoid arthritis
2. A-asbestosis
3. S-scleroderma
4. I-idiopathic
5. O-other
   - Busulphan, bleomycin, amiodarone, methotrexate

Diffuse Interstitial Disease + Mediastinal Lymphadenopathy

1. Carcinoma
2. Lymphoma
3. Sarcoidosis
4. Silicosis
5. Viral infection

Diffuse Interstitial Disease + Skeletal Abnormality

1. Ribs-scleroderma
2. Spine-ankylosing spondylitis
3. Shoulder joints-RA, scleroderma, sarcoidosis
   - Hypertrophic pulmonary osteoarthropathy
4. Skull-tuberous sclerosis, histiocytosis X

Miliary Opacities

1. Miliary pattern
   i. Sarcoidosis
   ii. Metastases-thyroid, renal, trophoblastic
   iii. TB
   iv. Silicosis
   v. Chickenpox
   vi. Fibrosing alveolitis
   vii. Pneumoconiosis
2. Dense nodules
   i. Silicosis
   ii. Chronic hemosiderosis
   iii. Metal
   iv. Microlithiasis

Cardiophrenic Angle Mass

1. Fat pad-obesity, lipoma, steroids
2. Hernia of Morgani
3. Pericardial cyst
4. Pericardial tumor

Hyperinflated Lungs

1. ***Bilateral hyperinflation***
   i. COAD
   ii. Asthma
   iii. α_1-antitrypsin deficiency
   iv. Cystic fibrosis
   v. Bronchiolitis
   vi. Aspergillosis

2. *Unilateral hyperinflation*
    i. Foreign body with hyperinflation
    ii. Pneumothorax
    iii. Large pulmonary embolus
    iv. Lung cyst, bullae
    v. Unilateral emphysema
    vi. Post-lobectomy hyperinflation
3. *Apparent unilateral hyperinflation*
    i. Rotated normal CXR
    ii. Increased density on other side
    iii. Absent breast
    iv. Absent pectoral muscle-congenital, surgical
    v. Scoliosis

Pulmonary Oligemia

1. Low cardiac output
2. R → L shunt-Fallot's, Ebstein's, triology
3. Pulmonary artery banding

Pulmonary Plethora

1. Features
    i. ≤ 1:1 distribution of vessel diameter-cf venous hypertension >1
    ii. Increase number of hilar vessels
2. Causes
    i. Hyperdynamic circulation-polycythemia
        - Thyrotoxicosis
        - Fluid overload

   ii. L→ R shunt-ASD, VSD, PDA
      - Partial anomalous pulmonary venous drainage
  iii. Bidirectional shunt-transposition, truncus arteriosus
      - Partial anomalous pulmonary venous drainage

Large Lesion on CXR

1. Common
    i. Tumor
   ii. Infection
  iii. TB
   iv. Hydatid
    v. Encased effusion
   vi. Progressive massive fibrosis
2. Uncommon
    i. Infection
   ii. Bronchogenic cyst
  iii. Pulmonary sequestration-aortic, not pulmonary
       artery supply
3. "Air-crescent" sign → cavity +
    i. Fungal infection
   ii. Clot
  iii. Tumor
   iv. Hydatid

Mediastinal Masses

1. *Commonest*
    i. Fat deposition—obesity, lipoma, steroids
   ii. Vascular

2. *Anterior*
   i. Thymus
   ii. Thyroid
   iii. Other tumor-teratoma, dermoid cyst, lipoma
   iv. Ascending aortic aneurysm
   v. Lymphadenopathy

3. *Middle*
   i. Heart
   ii. Aortic arch aneurysm
   iii. Pulmonary vessels
   iv. Trachea
   v. Bronchogenic cyst
   vi. Lymphadenopathy

4. *Posterior*
   i. Descending aortic aneurysm
   ii. Hiatus hernia
   iii. Diaphragmatic hernia
   iv. Lymphadenopathy
   v. Neuroma
   vi. Neuroblastoma
   vii. Enterogenic cyst

Calcification on CXR

1. *Localized calcification*
   i. Tuberculosis
   ii. Hematoma
   iii. Hamartoma-popcorn calcification
   iv. Teratoma
   v. Rarely-sarcoid, asbestosis

2. *Diffuse calcification*
    i. Post-varicella pneumonia
   ii. Tuberculosis
  iii. Histoplasmosis
   iv. Silicosis
    v. Chronic hemosiderosis

3. *Hilar calcification*
    i. Lymph nodes
       Tuberculosis
       Silicosis
       Sarcoidosis
       Histoplasmosis
   ii. Pulmonary atherosclerosis

4. *"eggshell" calcification*
    i. Silicosis
   ii. Sarcoid
  iii. Scleroderma
   iv. Anthracosis
    v. Lymphoma after radiotherapy
   vi. Amyloid
  vii. Histoplasmosis

5. *Pleural calcification*
    i. Tuberculosis
   ii. Empyema
  iii. Hemothorax
   iv. Asbestosis

Extrapleural Mass on CXR

1. Osteomyelitis

2. Actinomycosis
3. Hydatid
4. Tumor 1° or 2°
5. Myeloma
6. Fracture
7. Extramedullary hematopoiesis

Pleural Effusion

NB: > 300 ml
1. Loss of costophrenic angle
2. Upper border meniscus
3. Homogeneous opacity obscures heart border and diaphragm
4. Mediastinal shift
5. Increase distance between lung and stomach gas on left.
6. ***Lateral decubitus*** reveals change in meniscus and useful for small or unusual effusion

Massive Pleural Effusion

1. Post-thoracotomy/pneumonectomy
2. Tumor
3. Empyema
4. TB
5. Haemothorax
6. Ruptured oesophagus

Rib Notching

1. Coarctation of aorta

2. IVC obstruction
3. Neurofibromas
4. Tuberosclerosis
5. Idiopathic

CXR: Specific Pictures

Aspiration Pneumonitis

1. Normal CXR-small aspiration or too early
2. Linear (interstitial) densities
3. Nodular (alveolar) or patchy infiltrates
4. Lobar consolidation/collapse
5. Non-cardiogenic pulmonary edema (ARDS)

COPD

1. PA or AP
    i. Flattening of diaphragm
    ii. Thin heart shadow
    iii. Attenuation of vessels
    iv. Vessels "pulled" down → "like drooping moustache"
    v. Bullae
    vi. Bulging of lung edges → between ribs and around heart
2. Lateral
    i. Flattening of diaphragm
    ii. ↑ AP diameter
    iii. ↑ retrosternal air shadow
    iv. Bullae

3. Etiology
    i. Smoking
    ii. Chronic asthma
    iii. α_1-antitrypsin deficiency
    iv. Chronic dust/pollution exposure
    v. Cystic fibrosis

Sarcoidosis

1. Bilateral hilar lymphadenopathy
2. Opacities spreading from hilum into parenchyma
3. Miliary opacities-sarcoid nodules
4. Paratracheal lymphadenopathy

Tuberculosis

1. Unilateral hilar lymphadenopathy-1°TB
    ± calcification
2. Primary lesion in middle lobe or apex of lower lobe
3. Subapical lesion-opacity
    - cavity
    ± calcification
4. Bronchopneumonic changes
5. Miliary opacities-obscure normal lung markings
6. Acute lung injury, ARDS

Carcinoma

1. Possible CXR features,
    i. Consolidation/"pneumonia"
    ii. Apical mass ± rib erosion

   iii. Cavitating lesion
   iv. Lung abscess
   v. Lobar collapse
   vi. Paralysed hemidiaphragm
   vii. Hilar lymphadenopathy
  viii. Miliary shadowing from secondaries

2. **Lung metastases**
   i. Canon ball opacities
   ii. Miliary opacities
   iii. Numerous ill-defined opacities
   iv. Kerley B lines-obstructed lymphatics, no cardio-megaly

3. **Central mass** →
   i. Squamous ~ 40%
   ii. Anaplastic ~ 40% → large or small cell

4. **Peripheral mass** →
   i. Alveolar cell
   ii. Adenocarcinoma
   iii. Pancoast's

Pulmonary Embolus

1. Normal CXR
2. Transient unilateral increase in lung lucency
   Westermark's sign-due to generalized vasoconstriction
3. Unilateral peripheral translucent area
4. Pleurally-based, wedge-shaped or 'D'-shaped opacity on lateral CXR
   Hampton's hump
   Hazy opacity on PA CXR

5. Pleural effusion
6. Linear atelectasis
7. Raised hemidiaphragm
8. Enlargement of hilum
9. RV enlargement, azygos vein dilatation
10. Rarely calcification

Pulmonary Arterial Hypertension

1. Features
    i. Enlarged, well-defined hilar vessels-arise from hilum ± calcification
    ii. Rapid tapering of vessels
    iii. Very few peripheral vascular markings
    iv. No effusions or Kerley lines-i.e. no signs of LVF
    v. Cardiomegaly-RV and RA
    vi. Prominent IVC and SVC
    vii. CXR changes are *late*
2. Causes
    i. L → R shunt
    ii. Pulmonary embolism
    iii. Cor pulmonale
    iv. Mitral stenosis
    v. Idiopathic PAH

Pulmonary Venous Hypertension

1. Features = upper lobe venous diversion
    i. UL > LL veins
    ii. 1st interspace vessel > 3 mm

   iii. Any segmental artery > 5 mm
        NB: ↑ magnification on portable AP films, may
        exceed these limits
2. Causes
   i. LVF
   ii. Mitral stenosis
   iii. Left atrial-myxoma, tumor, thrombus
   iv. Cor triatriatum
   v. Anomalous pulmonary venous drainage
   vi. Constrictive pericarditis
   vii. Pulmonary venous fibrosis or thrombosis

Fat Embolus

1. Normal CXR in 88%
2. Patchy consolidation
3. Right heart failure
4. Bilateral diffuse infiltrates-ARDS

Lung Infiltrates in Renal Failure

1. Septicemia
2. Bacterial pneumonia
3. Cardiogenic shock
4. Acute lung injury
   i. ARDS
   ii. MOSF
5. Atypical pneumonia-*Legionella*
6. Autoimmune disease
   i. Goodpasteur's syndrome
   ii. Polyarteritis

iii. SLE
iv. Wegener's granulomatosis
7. Drug effects

Mesothelioma/Asbestosis

1. Exposure to asbestos fibers
2. Restrictive lung deficit
3. Radiological changes

CXR patterns of presentation,
a. Peripheral opacities
b. Geographical plaques and calcification
c. Pulmonary fibrosis
d. Bronchogenic carcinoma

Silicosis

1. Numerous small nodules—upper zones
2. Pulmonary fibrosis—upper zones
3. Egg-shell calcification—DDX sarcoid

Asbestosis Silicosis
- Interstitial fibrosis lower lobes upper lobes
- PMF uncommon common
- Malignancy mesothelioma
- Bronchogenic carcinoma
- Uncommon
- Tuberculosis uncommon common
- Calcification pleural lung, hilar nodes
- Respiratory failure common common
- Other features pleural thickening

- Pleural effusion
- Caplan's syndrome

CARDIAC

Heart Size

1. ***Small heart***
   i. Hyperinflated lungs-asthma, emphysema
   ii. Hypovolemia
   iii. Addison's disease
   iv. Cachexia, anorexia
   v. Normal variant
2. ***Massive enlargement***
   i. Mitral valve disease
   ii. Pericardial effusion
   iii. Cardiomyopathy
   iv. Ebstein's anomaly
3. ***Moderate enlargement*** → above plus,
   i. Ischemic heart disease
   ii. Hypertensive heart disease
   iii. Valvular heart disease
   iv. Cardiomyopathy
   v. Pericardial tumor, cyst
   vi. Factitious-supine or AP film
      - Raised hemidiaphragms
4. LA enlargement
   i. Mitral valve disease
   ii. LVF |
   iii. VSD | → pulmonary blood flow and LA volume
   iv. PDA | overload

Cardiac Failure CCF

1. Cardiomegaly
2. Pulmonary congestion $\rightarrow$ UL $\geq$ LL vessels
3. Prominent lymphatics
   i. Blurring of hilar vessels-dilated lymphatics
   ii. Visible lymphatics-Kerley A and B lines
4. Interstitial edema $\rightarrow$ reticular pattern, Kerley C lines
5. Alveolar edema
   i. Diffuse patchy opacities
   ii. "Cotton-wool" opacities around bronchi $\rightarrow$ LL > ML > UL
   iii. Blurring of cardiac borders
6. Pleural effusion, fluid in lobar fissures
   Lung fields reflect cardiac function better than heart size does.

Pulmonary Edema

1. ***Chronic/cardiogenic***
   i. Septal lines-Kerley's lines
   ii. Diffuse reticular pattern
   iii. Perivascular and peribronchial cuffing
   iv. Subpleural thickening and edema
   v. Perihilar and basal infiltrates
   vi. Upper lobe venous distension
   vii. Pleural effusion
   viii. Air bronchogram rare
2. ***Acute and/or non-cardiogenic-***e.g. ARDS
   i. Pathcy alveolar edema-not hilar

ii. Air bronchograms

iii. With well defined cardiac borders and

iv. No lymphatics nor venous congestion visible

v. Normal cardiac and PA size

Kerley's lines: A and B → septal lymphatics

A. Large, 4-6 cm, irregular, radiate from hilum to upper lobes

B. Short 1-2 cm, horizontal, basal, touch pleural margin
Transient—fluid
Permanent—MS, tumor, lymphangitis, pneumoconioses

C. Fine curvillinear, often generalized, giving reticular pattern.

Pulmonary Edema: Acute

NB: signs usually present in acute pulmonary edema, alveolar and interstitial edema with,

1. Normal heart size
2. Normal PA size
3. No venous congestion
4. Normal size azygos vein
5. Absence of Kerley's lines

Pulmonary Edema: Unilateral

1. Pulmonary embolus-on unaffected side
2. Re-expansion of collapsed lung or pneumothorax
3. Unilateral lung cysts or emphysema-on unaffected side
4. Severe cardiomegaly and CCF → R-sided edema (left PA compressed)

5. Patient in lateral position-gravity, dependant side
6. Aspiration pneumonitis
7. Congenital heart disease and shunt-e.g. Fallot's

Mitral Stenosis

1. Signs of high pulmonary venous pressure
   i. Kerly A & B septal lines
   ii. Prominent lesser fissure with fluid
   iii. Upper lobe venous distension
   iv. Pulmonary edema
   v. Dilated left atrium → see over
   vi. Straight left heart border and ↑ LA appendage
2. Other features
   i. Calcified mitral valve
   ii. Dilated pulmonary arteries > aortic diameter
   iii. ***Normal*** heart size in uncomplicated cases
       Undersized LV but abnormal function

Left Atrial Dilatation

1. PA or AP CXR
   i. Double heart border on right
   ii. Loss of LA appendage "trough"
   iii. Splayed carina
   iv. Cardiomegaly
   v. Esophageal displacement-NGT or barium swallow
   vi. ± pulmonary edema
2. Lateral CXR
   i. Posterior bulging of the cardiac border

Fallot's Tetralogy

1. Apex of the heart raised above level of hemidiaphragm
2. Pulmonary oligemia
3. Small pulmonary arteries
4. Dilated aorta

Atrial Septal Defect ASD

1. LA dilatation
2. RA dilatation
3. Large pulmonary artery
4. Dilated UL and LL veins
5. Small aortic arch < PA diameter
6. Septal defect with mongolism can → isolated RUL congestion (mechanism unknown)

Eisenmenger's Syndrome

Def'n: reversal of right → left shunt as a result of pulmonary hypertension
1. Large dilated main pulmonary arteries
2. Oligaemia of peripheral lung fields
3. Small aortic shadow

Coarctation of the Aorta

1. Rib notching → 3rd-7th ribs
2. "wasting" or "3-sign" on descending aorta-pre/post-stenotic dilatation
3. Prominent left subclavian artery
4. LAH
5. Cardiomegaly → LVH

Pericardial Effusion

NB: X-ray changes late $\rightarrow$ > 200 ml required

1. "Water-bag" cardiomegaly, large globular cardiac shadow
2. Acute angle between cardiac shadow and hemidiaphragms.
3. Clear heart border-no movement of heart seen to blurr film
4. Symmetrical cardiac enlargement
5. Clear lungs—no LVF

Constrictive Pericarditis

1. Cardiomegaly
2. Pericardial calcification-especially oblique and lateral
3. More common with,
   Chronic idiopathic
   Chronic renal failure
   Rheumatoid arthritis
   Neoplastic
   Tuberculosis
   Irradiation

Patent Ductus Arteriosus

1. 1-5 as for ASD
2. L atrial dilatation
3. R atrial dilatation
4. R ventricular dilatation
5. Large pulmonary artery
6. Dilated UL and LL veins
7. Large aorta

Right Heart Failure

1. Cardiomegaly-RV + RA
2. SVC and azygos vein distension
3. ± Pulmonary artery prominence
4. **No** alveolar edema

APPENDIX

CXR BASICS

REVIEW OF NORMAL CHEST

In many ways the skills needed to look at diagnostic radiographs are the same ones used for performing physical examinations on patients. For example, careful observation of findings coupled with a systematic review of systems are the same in both.

Get in the habit of always checking the following items before anything else. It takes a few seconds and is an important legal safe guard as well.

1. Patient's name.
2. Date exam done (very important if comparing prior exams).
3. Check for position markers-right vs. left, upright.

Other items to check before commencing with clinical review of the film include:

1. Patients position-supine, upright, lateral, decubitus.
2. Technical quality of exam-learn what are the acceptable limits for the exam. You can't find a subtle pneumothorax if there is patient motion or the film is overexposed.

INITIAL SURVEY

1. General Body Size, Shape, and Symmetry
2. Male vs. Female
3. Is this an infant, child, young adult, elderly person?
4. Survey for foreign objects-tubes, IV lines, ECG leads, surgical drains, prosthesis, etc. , as well as non-medical objects, bullets, shrapnel, glass, etc.

Soft Tissues and Skeletal Structure

Soft tissues-look again at overall amount, then check for the following: calcifications, obvious mass effect, abnormal air collections (called subcutaneous emphysema), and soft tissue companion shadow for the clavicle (this is a normal but variable finding).

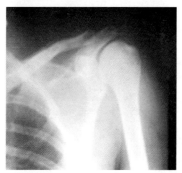

FIGURE 1: Shoulder girdle

Bones-look at each bone for the following items (notice again the progression from general to increasingly specific detail throughout the review).

1. Overall size, shape, and contour of each bone.
2. The density or mineralization.
3. Compare cortical thickness to medullary cavity, trabecular pattern, look for erosions, fractures, any lytic or blastic regions.
4. At joints, are articular relationships normal, joint spaces narrowed, widened, any calcification in the cartilages, air in the joint space, abnormal fat pads, etc.

CHEST WALL

Look for overall thickness, subcutaneous emphysema, calcification. Look for sharp, distinct borders.

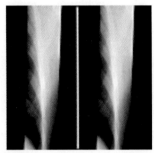

FIGURE 2: Chest wall with ribs

BREAST TISSUE

In males and females, some asymmetry can occur from standing with unequal pressure against the film holder. Notice how the apparent lung density changes from the lung area covered by the soft tissue of the breast to the lung area inferior to the breast.

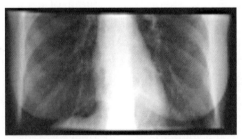

FIGURE 3: Breast shadow

ABDOMEN

The visibility of structures is highly variable but look for the following even if you see very few on any one exam.

1. Gastric and bowel gas—Is amount and location normal?
2. Check for organ size of liver, spleen, and kidneys if visible.
3. Check for free peritoneal air—Remember position of patient will change location of free air.
4. Look for calcifications and masses—Can they be localized to a specific structure.

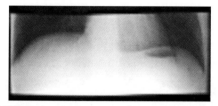

FIGURE 4: Diaphragm and gastric air bubble

NECK SOFT TISSUES AND SPINE

Check overall amounts of soft tissue, presence of calcifications, subcutaneous emphysema, position and size of

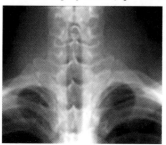

FIGURE 5: Neck—soft tissue, spine, accessory ribs

trachea. For the cervical spine, check alignment and note any major congenital abnormalities. Then look at specific parts of the vertebra and disk spaces, checking for erosions, lytic or blastic lesions, disk and synovial joint narrowing or other abnormalities.

THORACIC SPINE

Look at specific parts of each vertebra and the disk spaces as far caudally as the image allows, compare frontal and lateral projections. Some check list items to watch for are: height of vertebral bodies and disk spaces, integrity of cortical margins around the bodies, pedicles, and lamina, presence of any lytic or sclerotic areas, normal spacing of synovial joints, versus narrowing or sclerosis.

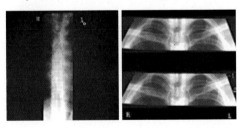

FIGURE 6: Thoracic spine, paravertebral stripes

RIBS

Compare individual ribs side to side, check specific parts, cortical margins, trabecular patterns. Make a note if the anterior cartilages are calcified, frequently the first one does so irregularly and may obscure or mimic underlying lung lesions.

1. Posterior rib
2. Anterior rib

SUPERIOR MEDIASTINUM-PA

First, check the overall width for normal size, again look for masses, calcifications, and free air. The rest of the superior mediastinum review is a detailed search for subtle distortion of several major pleural mediastinal interfaces.

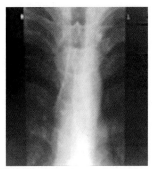

FIGURE 7: Superior mediastinal planes

MARGIN OF SUPERIOR VENA CAVA (SVC)

The SVC is seen on the frontal view only, and depending how laterally it projects, its right edge may cast a subtle line on the film. Sometimes the entire edge is seen, often only a portion, but it should not bulge into the lung with a convex border.

RIGHT PARATRACHEAL STRIPE

The normal width is less than 5 mm, usually it is only 2-3 mm. This is an important marker for otherwise subtle adenopathy. The distal end of the stripe is formed by the azygos vein, and if the vein is distended, that portion of the stripe may normally be up to 1 cm wide. The medial margin of the stripe is the air-soft tissue interface along the right mucosal surface of the trachea. The outer margin of the stripe begins around the level of the medial end of the clavicle and is formed by the pleural surface of the right upper lobe (RUL) against the mediastinum. The only structures normally at that level to give soft tissue density between the air filled trachea and the RUL are the right wall of the trachea, nerves, some fat, lymph nodes, and pleura of the RUL. The stripe ends where the RUL bronchus sweeps under the azygos vein as the latter arches anteriorly to empty into the posterior surface of the SVC.

LEFT SUBCLAVIAN STRIPE

The normal width is 1.0-1.5 cm. Its inner margin is the air mucosal interface along the left mucosal surface of the trachea, and its outer margin is the interface of the medial aspect of the left upper lobe against the lateral margin of the left subclavian artery. You usually will pick up the outer edge of the stripe at the level of the clavicle and will be able to follow it down to the bulge of the aortic arch.

Anterior Middle and Posterior Mediastinum

Review the heart for overall size and shape. A rough yardstick for size on the frontal film is the ratio of the widest diameter of the heart to the widest width of the thoracic cage as measured from inner aspect of rib to rib. This cardiac-thoracic ratio should be less than 50% (see inset for a graphic illustration of ratio measurements). Look carefully for calcifications, pneumopericardium, pneumomediastinum, sutures, prosthetic valves etc. , that you may have overlooked on the general survey of the entire mediastinum.

AORTA

Try tracking it from the root to distal descending aorta. In the young adult the ascending aorta usually is hidden in the mediastinum, in older people it may swing to the right enough to cast a soft tissue bulge. The arch should always be seen, make sure it is to the left of the distal trachea and actually pushes the distal trachea slightly to the right. Check for aortic calcifications and size. The left lateral border of the descending aorta abutts the left lung.

PULMONARY ARTERY

On the frontal view, the only part of the main pulmonary artery seen is the left lateral border where it meets the left lung. It can be relatively straight or convex (most commonly in young females). When convex, it forms a "middle mogul" just above the heart. The upper "mogul" is the aortic knob, the lower mogul is the left ventricle. The left pulmonary artery is directly behind the main pulmonary artery, and is visible on frontal films as a branching structure.

AZYGOSESOPHAGEAL LINE OR PARAESOPHAGEAL LINE

This is seen on the forntal view only and is formed by the right lower lobe where it meets the portion of the mediastinum containing the esophagus and the azygos vein. It usually overlies the thoracic spine, at or near the midline, and is usually fairly straight, vertically. If it bulges convex toward the lung, be suspicious of a mediastinal mass, usually subcarinal lymph nodes or an enlarged left atrium.

RIGHT AND LEFT PULMONARY ARTERIES

On the frontal view, the left pulmonary artery is the soft tissue density behind the main pulmonary artery, branching into the lung. The proximal right pulmonary artery is buried in the mediastinum, and is not seen on the frontal view until it branches as the right hilum.

PULMONARY ARTERIES, LATERAL VIEW

The right pulmonary artery is seen on the lateral view as an ovoid branching structure, just anterior to the air column of the trachea and main bronchi. The left pulmonary artery is never seen as clearly as the right, unless it is markedly enlarged. It is a curved shadow, similar in shape to the aorta, just behind the air column.

AORTICOPULMONARY WINDOW (AP WINDOW)

This is another area radiologists double check for subtle mediastinal masses. It is seen on the frontal view (line of white dots) and is formed by a portion of the upper lobe sitting in the space immediately lateral to the area between the aortic arch and left pulmonary artery (remember ligamentum arteriosum and left recurrent laryngeal nerve?). The AP window should have a concave or straight border. If there is a mediastinal mass in the AP window region, the lung will be pushed laterally and the border becomes convex.

PARASPINAL EDGES (STRIPES)

Sometimes on the frontal view, the pleural edge is seen as a vertical density running parallel to the lateral margins of the vertebral bodies. If visible, this edge should be only a few millimeters beyond the vertebral bodies, and should not be lumpy or bulging. (The paraspinal edges are not visible on this image.)

HILA

FRONTAL VIEW OF THE HILA

As visible on the frontal view, most of the hilar shadows are the left and right pulmonary arteries. The bronchi run with the arteries, but are, of course, lucent. The pulmonary veins are not clearly seen because they are behind the widest parts of the heart, inferior to the hila, where they converge into the left atrium. The left pulmonary artery is always more superior than the right, thus making the left hilum appear higher. Calcified lymph nodes may be visible within the hilar shadows.

PARENCHYMA

Large abnormalities will have already been seen, but now is the time to search carefully for small masses, infiltrates, calcifications, etc. Compare small sections of lung side to side at a time. Use the same techniques as you used for comparing ribs but now ignore the bone and look at the lung. There are three areas in which small lung lesions are easily overlooked: behind the calcified anterior first rib cartilage, behind the heart, and behind the diaphragm.

LATERAL VIEW OF THE LUNG

The lateral view is your great chance to look at the lung in the posterior costophrenic recess and anterior mediastinum.

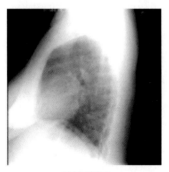

FIGURE 8

Pleura

Check the frontal view for minor fissure thickness and location, and on the lateral view, look for minor and major fissures even if you do not see them in their entirety which you rarely will. These are normally fine delicate structures that do not show up on the digitized images.

Check List

1. Check patient name, position, technical quality.
2. Soft tissue including breast, chest wall, companion shadow.
3. Review soft tissues and skeletal structures of shoulder girdles and chest wall.
4. Review abdomen for bowel gas, organ size, abnormal calcifications, free air, etc.
5. Review soft tissues and spine of neck.
6. Review spine and rib cage: check alignment, disk space narrowing, lytic or blastic regions, etc.
7. Review mediastinum:
   A. Overall size and shape
   B. Trachea: position
   C. Margins: SVC, ascending aorta, right atrium, left subclavian artery, aortic arch, main pulmonary artery, left ventricle
   D. Lines and stripes: paratracheal, paraspinal, para-esophageal (azygosesophageal), paraaortic
   E. Retrosternal clear space
8. Review hila:
   A. Normal relationships
   B. Size
9. Review lungs and pleura:
   A. Compare lung sizes

B. Evaluate pulmonary vascular pattern: compare upper to lower lobe, right to left, normal tapering to periphery

C. Pulmonary parenchyma

D. Pleural surfaces

   a. Fissures-major and minor-if seen

   b. Compare hemidiaphragms

   c. Follow pleura around rib cage.

INDEX